WALL PILATES WORKOUTS FOR WOMEN

CLAUDIA LYNNE

RMC PUBLISHERS

CONTENTS

INTRODUCTION

Are you tired of fitness programs that promise the world but deliver little? Have you struggled to find an exercise routine that fits seamlessly into your busy life? Do you long for a workout that not only strengthens your body and helps you lose weight but also works to balance your mind and body?

Wall Pilates is a revolutionary approach to fitness that combines the core-strengthening principles of traditional Pilates with the stability and resistance provided by a simple wall. This unique method offers a full-body workout that builds strength, improves flexibility, enhances your mind-body connection, and aids in weight loss—all without expensive equipment or gym memberships.

Wall Pilates Workouts for Women has been crafted to provide you with the tools you need to begin your transformative fitness journey. In just 10 minutes a day, you can build lean muscle, balance stress hormones, and shed fat.

The power of wall Pilates lies in its ability to engage multiple muscle groups simultaneously while promoting proper alignment and posture. When using the wall as your prop, you can perform exercises with greater stability and control, making it an ideal practice for people of all fitness levels. The mind-body connection fostered with each wall Pilates exercise helps build physical strength, reduce stress, improve focus, and boost your body's ability to lose weight without long, intense workouts. Recent studies have shown that mind-body exercises like wall Pilates can significantly improve physical function, reduce pain, and enhance quality of life (Yamato et al., 2015).

Each week of your wall Pilates workout plan will introduce you to targeted exercises that gradually increase in intensity. Throughout the chapters to come, you will:

- Be introduced to wall Pilates and why it benefits weight loss, strength training, and building a lean, agile body.
- Learn how to set up your own workout area to maximize each of your 10-minute workouts.
- Be provided step-by-step instructions for each exercise, complete with clear illustrations.
- Learn progressive workout routines to guide you through your 28-day weight loss journey.

Introduction

- Be taught breathing techniques to enhance your mind-body connection and activate your body's natural weight loss systems.
- Be provided with a 28-day meal plan to support your fitness goals.
- Learn modifications and alternatives for each exercise so that your wall Pilates workouts can meet you where you are on your fitness journey.

Combining wall Pilates's physical exercise and mindfulness practices is a powerful tool for overall well-being. Whether you're a fitness novice looking for an accessible entry-point workout or an experienced exerciser looking for ways to diversify your routine, wall Pilates offers a simple path to strength, flexibility, and health. By the end of this 28-day journey, you'll have all the tools to continue your wall Pilates practice independently, adapting it to your evolving needs and goals.

Are you ready to discover the transformative power of wall Pilates? Let's begin this journey together, one breath and one movement at a time.

CHAPTER 1
UNDERSTANDING WALL PILATES

*A*re you ready to revolutionize your fitness routine and unlock the power of Pilates without the need for expensive equipment or gym memberships? Pilates has already revolutionized the lives of hundreds of thousands of people since the early 1900s.

For you to understand what wall Pilates is, we first need to uncover how it was developed and what the aim of this powerful, low-impact workout is.

Joseph Pilates, the visionary behind this transformative workout, was dedicated to creating a method that strengthened the core, improved posture, and nurtured the vital connection between mind and body. He recognized the profound impact our thoughts, emotions, and beliefs can have on our physical well-being. Pilates became the physical manifestation of Joseph's interest in the strength of the human body when fitness was approached holistically.

Pilates evolved over time, developed initially to be completed in small spaces or on specialized equipment called a reformer. While the traditional Pilates reformer exercises are undeniably effective, they are not always practical for those with limited space or budget. Wall Pilates was borne out of an adaptation of the core principles of Pilates, using the one piece of equipment almost everyone has access to —a wall. With this ingenious modification, you can achieve the same core-strengthening, posture-enhancing benefits of Pilates without costly equipment or studio memberships.

Don't be fooled into thinking that wall Pilates is a watered-down version of traditional Pilates practices. In fact, many Pilates devotees find that incorporating the wall into their practice intensifies their workouts. This is because the wall provides extra support and feedback, allowing you to focus on proper alignment and engagement in a way that can be more challenging to achieve on the mat alone.

The Principles of Pilates

Pilates operates on six fundamental principles. Each principle is designed to work together to create a workout that not only sculpts and strengthens your body but also nurtures your mind and spirit.

Let's explore each one in detail:

1. **Control:** In Pilates, every movement is executed with intention and precision. By engaging your muscles deliberately and purposefully, you'll develop a deep sense of control over your body, allowing you to move with grace and power.
2. **Centering:** Pilates's focal point is your core. By keeping your movements centered around your midline, you'll cultivate a stronger, more stable foundation that will make every exercise feel effortless and invigorating.
3. **Concentration:** Pilates is not just a physical practice; it's a mental one, too. Bringing your full attention and focus to each movement allows you to create a meditation session for your body and mind, leaving you feeling centered, calm, and energized.
4. **Precision:** In Pilates, quality trumps quantity every time. Paying meticulous attention to the smallest details ensures that you execute each movement accurately, ensuring maximum benefit and minimal risk of injury.
5. **Breathing:** Deep, purposeful breathing is the key to unlocking the full potential of your Pilates practice. Oxygenating your muscles and moving with each breath allows you to experience a newfound sense of ease, fluidity, and vitality in every movement.
6. **Flow:** Pilates is a dance between your body and your breath, seamlessly transitioning from one movement to another. By cultivating a sense of flow in your practice, you'll maximize your calorie burn without requiring lengthy or strenuous workouts.

Incorporating these six principles into your Pilates practice empowers you to transform your body and mind—unlocking a stronger, more balanced, and vibrant you.

Adaptation of Pilates for the Wall

There are several differences between traditional Pilates and wall Pilates. Traditional Pilates generally requires more balance and stability, deeply engaging the core. Concentrating on balance can often result in less attention being paid to form.

With wall Pilates, however, the wall acts as support and can guide you to align your body correctly. This ensures you complete each movement precisely, maximizing your time in just 10 minutes.

The wall provides extra assistance and feedback, helping you maintain proper form and engagement throughout every movement. Wall Pilates also offers a unique level of versatility you do not experience with traditional reformer work. Using the wall as a prop, you will discover a new range of movements and angles that are not possible when working on a reformer or the mat.

These subtle changes in alignment also present you with greater resistance, making it easier to feel when your body is out of alignment and intensify your workout.

With heightened awareness, you can correct learned poor posture issues, correct imbalances in your body, and begin strengthening muscles that have been working incorrectly.

Pilates and the Importance of Breath

Intentional, purposeful breathing is critical for a proper wall Pilates workout. Not only does breathing strengthen the mind-body connection, but it also ensures that your muscles are fully fueled as you move through each exercise. Well-oxygenated muscles are efficient muscles that will keep you balanced, strong, and energized throughout our wall Pilates routines.

While there are many conscious breathing practices, one is particularly effective for wall Pilates—lateral thoracic breathing.

Lateral Thoracic Breathing

This powerful form of conscious breathing allows you to fill your lungs with air during inhalation. The movement and core engagement involved in lateral thoracic breathing further engage your core, ensuring your abdominal muscles remain activated throughout your workout. Here's how to begin practicing lateral thoracic breathing.

- Begin your practice sessions by finding a comfortable sitting or lying position.
- Place your hands on your ribcage just below your armpits.
- Inhale deeply through your nose and concentrate on spreading your ribcage laterally—you will feel the expansion of your lungs as your ribcage grows under your hands.
- Using your core muscles, bring your belly button in toward your spine as you release the breath.
- Repeat five times, paying attention to how your rib cage expands and contracts with each breath in and out.

Continue to practice your lateral breathing, aiming to increase your repetitions from 5 to 8. Once you can comfortably achieve eight lateral breaths, you are ready to begin your wall Pilates exercises. In the meantime, while you practice your conscious breathing, let's look at how you can adequately prepare for the other aspects of your 28-day wall Pilates challenge.

CHAPTER 2
PREPARING FOR YOUR WALL PILATES PRACTICE

*P*reparing for your wall Pilates journey ensures you can transform not just your body but your mind and outlook on health and fitness. By optimizing your surroundings and fueling your body correctly, you are setting yourself up for success in your workouts.

Preparing Your Body for Your 28-Day Transformation Challenge

Before continuing with this section, I'd like to remind you that success is rarely linear, nor is it a cookie-cutter approach. The goals you set for yourself are personal, and while you will be guided through these 28 days, your workout routine and diet do not need to strictly follow what has been set out for you.

It's perfectly acceptable to take time to learn a particular move or concept and slow things down; you're not in competition with anybody here.

Your 28-Day Meal Plan

Below is a 28-day meal plan to help you nourish your body, enjoy your meals, and support your weight loss journey. Our team's certified holistic nutritionist thoughtfully created this plan. However, remember that individual preferences, dislikes, or food allergies may require adjustments. For detailed recipes accompanying this meal plan, please refer to the end of this book.

Week 1

Day 1
Breakfast: Superfood Smoothie Bowl
Lunch: Mediterranean Quinoa Salad
Snack: Apple Slices with Almond Butter
Dinner: Grilled Salmon with Asparagus

Day 2
Breakfast: Avocado Toast with Poached Egg
Lunch: Turkey and Avocado Wrap
Snack: Carrot Sticks and Hummus
Dinner: Slow Cooker Turkey Chili

Day 3
Breakfast: Greek Yogurt Parfait
Lunch: Veggie-Packed Frittata
Snack: Homemade Trail Mix
Dinner: Zucchini Noodles with Pesto and Chicken

Day 4
Breakfast: Avocado Toast with Poached Egg
Lunch: Mediterranean Quinoa Salad
Snack: Carrot Sticks and Hummus
Dinner: Slow Cooker Turkey Chili

Day 5
Breakfast: Superfood Smoothie Bowl
Lunch: Veggie-Packed Frittata
Snack: Apple Slices with Almond Butter
Dinner: Zucchini Noodles with Pesto and Chicken

Day 6
Breakfast: Greek Yogurt Parfait
Lunch: Turkey and Avocado Wrap
Snack: Homemade Trail Mix
Dinner: Grilled Salmon with Asparagus

Day 7
Breakfast: Superfood Smoothie Bowl
Lunch: Veggie-Packed Frittata
Snack: Carrot Sticks and Hummus
Dinner: Slow Cooker Turkey Chili

Week 2

Day 1
Breakfast: Overnight Oats with Berries
Lunch: Caprese Salad with Grilled Chicken
Snack: Hard-Boiled Eggs with Everything Bagel Seasoning
Dinner: Spaghetti Squash with Marinara and Meatballs

Day 2
Breakfast: Breakfast Burrito
Lunch: Tuna Salad Lettuce Wraps
Snack: Cucumber Slices with Cream Cheese and Smoked Salmon
Dinner: Sheet Pan Chicken Fajitas

Day 3
Breakfast: Peanut Butter Banana Smoothie
Lunch: Harvest Grain Bowl
Snack: Roasted Chickpeas with Cumin and Smoked Paprika
Dinner: Lentil and Vegetable Curry

Day 4
Breakfast: Breakfast Burrito
Lunch: Caprese Salad with Grilled Chicken
Snack: Roasted Chickpeas with Cumin and Smoked Paprika
Dinner: Lentil and Vegetable Curry

Day 5
Breakfast: Peanut Butter Banana Smoothie
Lunch: Tuna Salad Lettuce Wraps
Snack: Hard-Boiled Eggs with Everything Bagel Seasoning
Dinner: Sheet Pan Chicken Fajitas

Day 6
Breakfast: Overnight Oats with Berries
Lunch: Harvest Grain Bowl
Snack: Cucumber Slices with Cream Cheese and Smoked Salmon
Dinner: Spaghetti Squash with Marinara and Meatballs

Day 7
Breakfast: Peanut Butter Banana Smoothie
Lunch: Caprese Salad with Grilled Chicken
Snack: Roasted Chickpeas with Cumin and Smoked Paprika
Dinner: Sheet Pan Chicken Fajitas

Week 3

Day 1
Breakfast: Chia Seed Pudding with Mango
Lunch: Greek Salad with Grilled Shrimp
Snack: Celery Sticks with Peanut Butter and Raisins
Dinner: Baked Cod with Tomato-Olive Relish

Day 2
Breakfast: Savory Breakfast Bowl
Lunch: Veggie-Hummus Wrap
Snack: Greek Yogurt with Honey and Walnuts
Dinner: Stuffed Portobello Mushrooms

Day 3
Breakfast: Chocolate-Banana Protein Pancakes
Lunch: Pesto Chicken Salad
Snack: Homemade Kale Chips
Dinner: Turkey-Zucchini Meatballs with Spaghetti

Day 4
Breakfast: Savory Breakfast Bowl
Lunch: Greek Salad with Grilled Shrimp
Snack: Homemade Kale Chips
Dinner: Turkey-Zucchini Meatballs with Spaghetti

Day 5
Breakfast: Chocolate-Banana Protein Pancakes
Lunch: Veggie-Hummus Wrap
Snack: Celery Sticks with Peanut Butter and Raisins
Dinner: Baked Cod with Tomato-Olive Relish

Day 6
Breakfast: Chia Seed Pudding with Mango
Lunch: Pesto Chicken Salad
Snack: Greek Yogurt with Honey and Walnuts
Dinner: Stuffed Portobello Mushrooms

Day 7
Breakfast: Chocolate-Banana Protein Pancakes
Lunch: Greek Salad with Grilled Shrimp
Snack: Homemade Kale Chips
Dinner: Baked Cod with Tomato-Olive Relish

Week 4

Day 1
Breakfast: Sweet Potato Toast with Avocado
Lunch: Mason Jar Cobb Salad
Snack: Cherry Tomatoes with Mozzarella and Basil
Dinner: Grilled Steak with Chimichurri

Day 2
Breakfast: Blueberry-Almond Smoothie Bowl
Lunch: Curried Chicken Salad
Snack: Sliced Pear with Blue Cheese and Walnuts
Dinner: Quinoa-Stuffed Bell Peppers

Day 3
Breakfast: Egg and Veggie Muffins
Lunch: Veggie-Packed Minestrone Soup
Snack: Homemade Hummus with Veggie Sticks
Dinner: Shrimp Stir-Fry with Brown Rice

Day 4
Breakfast: Blueberry-Almond Smoothie Bowl
Lunch: Mason Jar Cobb Salad
Snack: Homemade Hummus with Veggie Sticks
Dinner: Quinoa-Stuffed Bell Peppers

Day 5
Breakfast: Egg and Veggie Muffins
Lunch: Curried Chicken Salad
Snack: Cherry Tomatoes with Mozzarella and Basil
Dinner: Shrimp Stir-Fry with Brown Rice

Day 6
Breakfast: Sweet Potato Toast with Avocado
Lunch: Veggie-Packed Minestrone Soup
Snack: Sliced Pear with Blue Cheese and Walnuts
Dinner: Grilled Steak with Chimichurri

Day 7
Breakfast: Egg and Veggie Muffins
Lunch: Mason Jar Cobb Salad
Snack: Cherry Tomatoes with Mozzarella and Basil
Dinner: Quinoa-Stuffed Bell Peppers

Setting Up a Designated Area for Wall Pilates

Once your body is fueled correctly, you can create your dedicated wall Pilates space. While not strictly required, taking the time to set up a designated area that's both functional and beautiful will help keep you motivated and looking forward to your next workout.

Choosing the Right Wall

- Select a wall at least two feet above your height to ensure ample space for a full range of motion. For example, if you're 5'6", opt for a wall at least 7'6" long.
- Ensure you have at least 6 feet of floor space to accommodate lateral movements and experimentation with different postures and angles.
- An 8- to 9-foot wall in height should be sufficient to perform all the exercises.
- Ensure the wall is free from any windows, doors, furniture, or artwork that might obstruct your practice or prevent you from direct contact with the wall surface.

Optimizing Lighting and Ventilation

- While many people prefer a dimly lit space for better concentration, choosing an area with ample natural light or good overhead lighting is essential to stay alert, focused, and aware of one's form and alignment.
- Ensure your wall Pilates area has proper ventilation and a cool temperature to keep you comfortable and energized throughout your workouts.

Selecting the Best Flooring

- Choose a hard floor with some traction, such as hardwood or tile, to provide a stable and supportive foundation for your practice.
- If your home is fully carpeted, consider investing in a high-quality yoga mat to create a firm, non-slip surface for your movements.

Working with Different Wall Materials

- Drywall, the most common wall material in modern American homes, is generally sturdy enough for gentle wall Pilates pressure and resistance. However, exercise caution and avoid excessive force or weight, especially in vulnerable areas like corners or seams.
- When using wooden walls, place a yoga mat or towel between your body and the wall to minimize the risk of scratches and scuffs.
- Brick walls offer the ultimate durability and resilience, capable of handling even the most enthusiastic wall Pilates sessions with ease.

Creating a Sacred Space

- Clear your wall Pilates area of clutter, noise, or distractions so your environment encourages focus, concentration, and inner peace.

- Bring personal touches into your workout space. This can include vibrant artwork, lush plants, or a soothing essential oil diffuser.

By thoughtfully designing your wall Pilates sanctuary, you'll create a space that supports your physical practice and nurtures your mind and spirit. As you step into this workout area each day, take a moment to set an intention, connect with your breath, and open yourself to the potential that lies within you.

With your wall Pilates space now ready, let's examine some equipment that can modify and enhance your workouts.

Equipment and How to Use it Effectively

The beauty of wall Pilates lies in its simplicity and the ability to give your body a full workout without equipment. That said, incorporating a few key pieces of equipment can enhance your experience and help you achieve even greater results.

Wall and Mat

- Although the wall may not be considered traditional equipment, it's the cornerstone of your practice. Ensure you have a sturdy, smooth wall free from obstructions and provide ample space for your movements.
- Invest in a high-quality yoga mat to cushion and support your joints while keeping you stable and grounded throughout your exercises.

Resistance Bands

- While entirely optional, resistance bands are a versatile and portable way to add challenge and intensity to your wall Pilates routine.
- Start with three bands: light, medium, and heavy. This will allow you to progressively challenge yourself and target specific muscle groups as you grow stronger and more comfortable with your practice.
- For wall Pilates, a 5-foot band is a good starting point. It provides ample room to maneuver and adjust resistance levels without feeling cumbersome. Taller individuals or those with longer limbs may prefer a slightly longer band.

Hand Weights

- Incorporating light hand weights (1-3 pounds) is an excellent way to boost your upper body strength and add an extra dimension to your wall Pilates workouts.
- Hand weights are optional, and proper form and alignment must be prioritized before adding external resistance.

Foam Rollers

- While not strictly necessary, foam rollers can be incredible for releasing tension, improving flexibility, and promoting muscle recovery before and after your wall Pilates sessions.
- Incorporating foam rolling into your routine'll help your body move more freely and efficiently, enhancing your overall Pilates experience.

Investing in these simple yet effective tools and learning to use them mindfully ensures you are well-equipped for your workouts. As you progress through your 28-day program, trust in the power of your body, the support of your equipment, and the transformative potential of this incredible practice.

Safety Considerations

As you begin with your wall Pilates journey, it's crucial to remember that your safety and well-being should always come first. While this wall Pilates offers a wealth of incredible benefits, it's essential to approach it with mindfulness, caution, and a deep respect for your body's unique needs and limitations.

Proper Form and Alignment

- Proper form and alignment are at the heart of a safe and effective wall Pilates practice. By maintaining optimal alignment of your musculoskeletal system, you'll get the most out of each exercise and minimize the risk of injury (Agnes, 2023).
- Focus on keeping your core engaged, your spine neutral, and your movements controlled and precise throughout each session.
- To find your neutral spine, imagine your body from the side, with a straight line passing downwards through your ears, shoulders, hips, knees, and ankles. Avoid excessive arching or rounding in any part of your spine.
- Achieve a neutral pelvis by ensuring your hip bones point straight ahead and your pubic bone aligns with your belly button. Gently rock your pelvis forward and backward until you find the sweet spot where these landmarks are in the same plane.

Leveraging the Wall for Alignment

- One remarkable advantage of wall Pilates is that the wall itself is a valuable tool for maintaining proper alignment.
- As you progress through your practice, continue using the wall as a guide and reference point, making adjustments to ensure optimal form and alignment.

Choosing Appropriate Exercises for Your Fitness Level

- While it may be tempting to dive headfirst into the most challenging wall Pilates exercises, it's crucial to start with a solid foundation of basic movements and gradually progress as your strength and skill develop.

- Remember that even the simplest exercises can be more challenging if you focus on proper form, engagement, and breath.
- Trust in the process and honor your body's unique journey. With consistent practice and dedication, you can safely and effectively advance your wall Pilates practice over time.

Listening to Your Body's Signals

- Above all, cultivate a deep sense of body awareness and respect for your individual needs and limitations.
- If, at any point during your practice, you experience sharp pain, shooting sensations, or a feeling that something isn't quite right, stop immediately and reassess.

Keep these safety considerations at the forefront of your mind and approach your wall Pilates journey with mindfulness and care, and you'll be well-equipped to reap the rewards of this transformative practice—Let's begin.

CHAPTER 3
WARMING-UP

*W*arming up is a critical element of any workout. The American Council on Exercise advises, "A well-rounded warm-up routine can help to gradually increase your heart rate, improve blood flow, and prepare your muscles and joints for the upcoming activity" (Cronkleton, 2019).

The warm-up exercises below are designed to gradually awaken your muscles, lubricate your joints, and get your blood pumping in preparation for the full workouts ahead.

As you move through your warm-up, focus on your breath, allowing it to guide and deepen each movement. Inhale as you prepare, exhale as you engage, and let the rhythm of your breath set the tempo for your entire practice.

Warm-Up Exercises

Leg Swings

Leg Swings improve hip mobility, enhance dynamic flexibility, and warm up the lower body muscles.

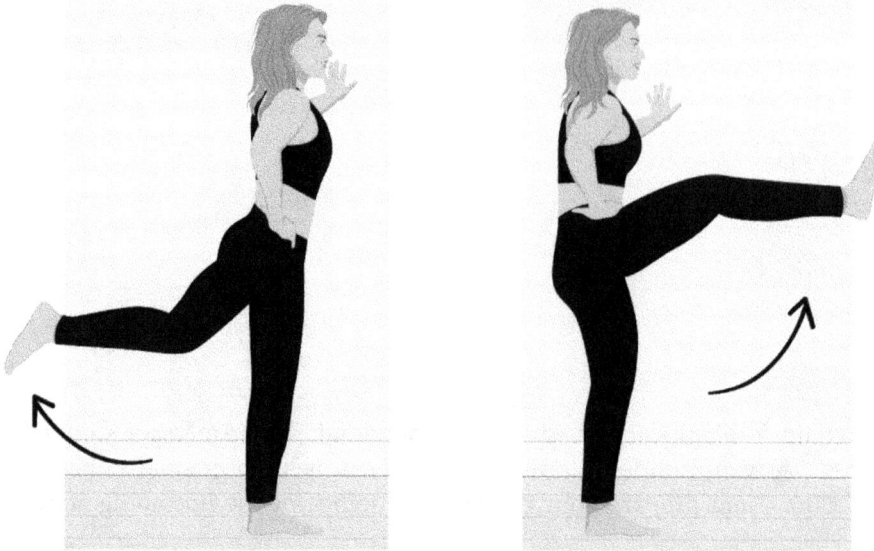

Instructions

- Stand next to a wall, with your left side facing the wall.
- Shift your weight onto your left leg, which will be your standing leg.
- Keep your right leg straight but not locked; swing it forward and backward with control.
- Start with small swings and gradually increase the range of motion as you warm up.
- Keep your upper body stable and facing forward throughout the movement.
- Perform front-to-back swings for 15 seconds.
- Turn around so that your right side is facing the wall.
- Swing your left leg front-to-back for 15 seconds.

Modifications

- Easier: Reduce the range of motion and focus on controlled smaller swings.
- Harder: Increase the speed of the swings while maintaining control or perform the exercise without holding onto the wall for support.
- Props: Use a resistance band around your ankles to engage stabilizing muscles.

Tips

- Keep your core engaged throughout the exercise to maintain balance and protect your back.
- Breathe naturally and rhythmically as you swing.
- Maintain a slight bend in your standing leg to avoid locking the knee.

Hip Twists

Hip Twists use the wall to improve core strength, enhance spinal mobility, and target obliques.

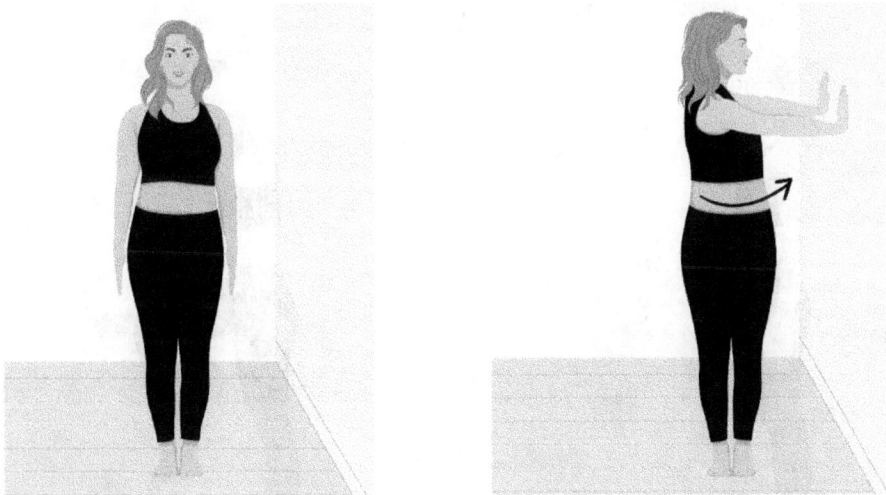

Instructions

- Stand with your right side facing a wall, about an arm's length away.
- Place your right palm flat against the wall at shoulder height for support.
- Keep your toes pointing forward.
- Engage your core and maintain a neutral spine.
- Keeping both feet planted firmly, rotate your upper body to the right, toward the wall.
- As you twist, allow your left arm to reach across your body, and if you can, place your left hand on the wall.
- Hold the twist for 15 seconds, feeling the stretch in your obliques and lower back.
- Slowly return to the starting position.
- Turn around so your left side faces the wall and repeat the exercise.

Modifications

- Easier: Stand closer to the wall and perform smaller twists, focusing on control.
- Harder: Step further away from the wall, using less support from your hand. You can also rise onto the balls of your feet as you twist for an added balance challenge.
- Props: Use a yoga strap or resistance band held taut between both hands to increase upper-body engagement.

Tips

- Focus on lengthening your spine upward as you twist, avoiding any slumping or leaning.

Standing Knee to Chest

Standing Knee to Chest with a wall provides improved hip flexibility and lower back stretching while offering additional stability.

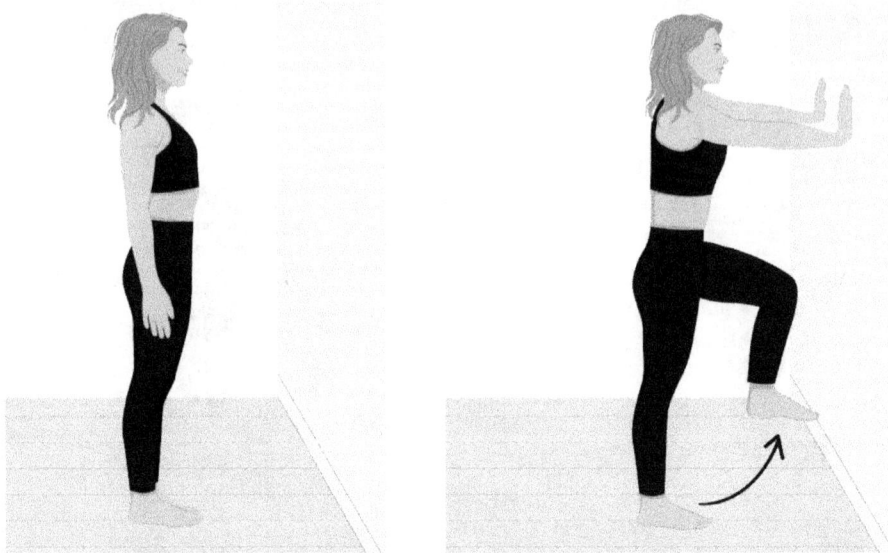

Instructions

- Stand facing a wall, about an arm's length away.
- Place your palms flat against the wall at chest height for support.
- Stand with your feet together and engage your core.
- Slowly lift your left knee toward your chest, keeping your right leg slightly bent.
- Hold this position for 15 seconds, breathing deeply and steadily.
- Slowly lower your left foot back to the ground.
- Repeat on the other side, lifting your right knee toward your chest.

Modifications

- Easier: Stand closer to the wall and use both hands on the wall for support if needed.
- Harder: Hold the knee-to-chest position for longer, or add a slight twist by pulling your knee towards the opposite shoulder.
- Props: Use a small towel or yoga strap to help you pull your knee closer.

Tips

- Keep your spine neutral, and avoid leaning forward or arching your back.
- Engage your abdominal muscles to support your lower back throughout the movement.
- Breathe deeply, exhaling as you pull your knee in and inhaling as you release.
- If you feel any strain in your lower back, reduce the range of motion or hold your leg lower on the thigh.

Cat-Cow

Cat-Cow improves spinal flexibility, strengthens the core, and helps relieve back tension.

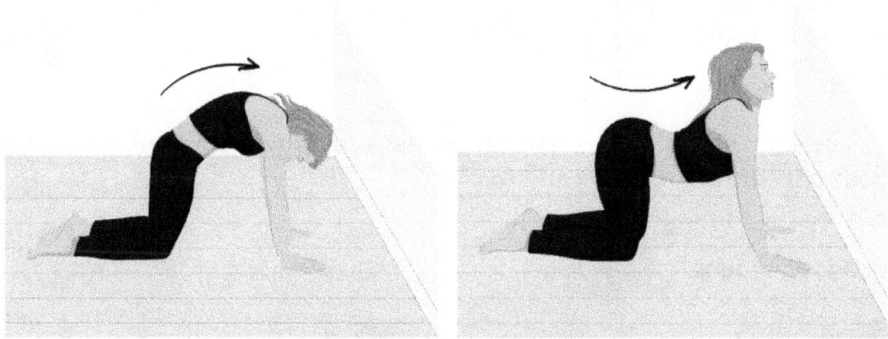

Instructions

- Start on your hands and knees in a tabletop position.
- Place your hands directly under your shoulders and knees under your hips.
- Keep your spine neutral and your head looking down at the floor.
- As you inhale, drop your belly towards the mat, lift your chin and chest, and gaze up toward the ceiling. This is Cow pose.
- Draw your shoulders away from your ears and feel the stretch in your abdomen.
- Exhale and round your spine to the ceiling, tucking your chin to your chest. This is Cat pose.
- Pull your navel toward your spine and feel the stretch in your back.
- Continue this flowing movement, matching your breath to each movement.
- Inhale for Cow, exhale for Cat.
- Repeat for 30 seconds.

Modifications

- Easier: Perform smaller movements, focusing on breath and subtle spinal flexion and extension.
- Harder: Add arm and leg extensions. Extend one arm forward and the opposite leg back in the Cow pose. Return to neutral before moving to the Cat pose.
- Props: Place a folded blanket under your knees for extra cushioning if you have sensitive knees.

Tips

- Keep your movements slow and controlled, synchronizing them with your breath.
- Maintain the distance between your hands and knees throughout the exercise.
- Focus on moving your spine vertebra by vertebra.
- If you have neck issues, keep your gaze between your hands instead of looking up in a Cow pose.
- Avoid letting your elbows lock; keep a micro-bend in them.

WALL PILATES WORKOUTS FOR WOMEN

Warm-Up Routine

1. Leg Swings: 15 seconds on each side.
2. Hip Twists: 15 seconds on each side.
3. Standing Knee to Chest: 15 seconds on each side.
4. Cat-Cow: 30 seconds

Now that you've done the essential warm-up exercises, let's continue with week 1, where we'll begin with the foundations of your wall Pilates workout.

Access to Instructional Videos

Thank you for choosing my book!
Enjoy exclusive access to instructional videos for every pose in the 28-day program by scanning the QR code below with your phone camera.
A link will appear. Tap the link, and it will take you to the videos.

https://youtube.com/playlist?list=PLdhFR3wj4TZjxS6js_gmso0iWjz7Nvaxy&si=KsRaR0Mtqpnjf6-l

CHAPTER 4
WEEK 1—FOUNDATION PILATES WORKOUT

*W*eek one introduces the fundamental movements needed to strengthen your core and align your posture. While you may feel tempted to start with more challenging exercises, these foundational movements are specifically designed to provide you with a strong foundation for your body to become stronger.

Concentrating on these fundamental steps will firmly position you to achieve your fitness and weight loss goals as you develop body awareness and a mind-muscle connection.

Focusing on Building Core Strength and Stability

"Core strength" refers to the group of muscles around your pelvis, lower back, hips, and stomach. These include all of your abdominal muscles. A strong core helps prevent injuries like a runner's knee or hip bursitis by improving support of the joints around these areas. In other words, your core is the central powerhouse of your entire body. It's the foundation that supports every movement, every breath, and every wall Pilates pose you will do in the coming weeks.

Day 1 to 4: Foundational Wall Pilates Exercises

As you begin your first week's exercises, remember to focus on proper form, alignment, and breath. The goal is not to perform a large number of repetitions but rather to ensure your muscles are engaging and that you're moving comfortably.

Wall Plank

Wall Planks strengthen the core, improve posture, and engage the shoulders and back muscles. This exercise is excellent for building isometric strength and stability.

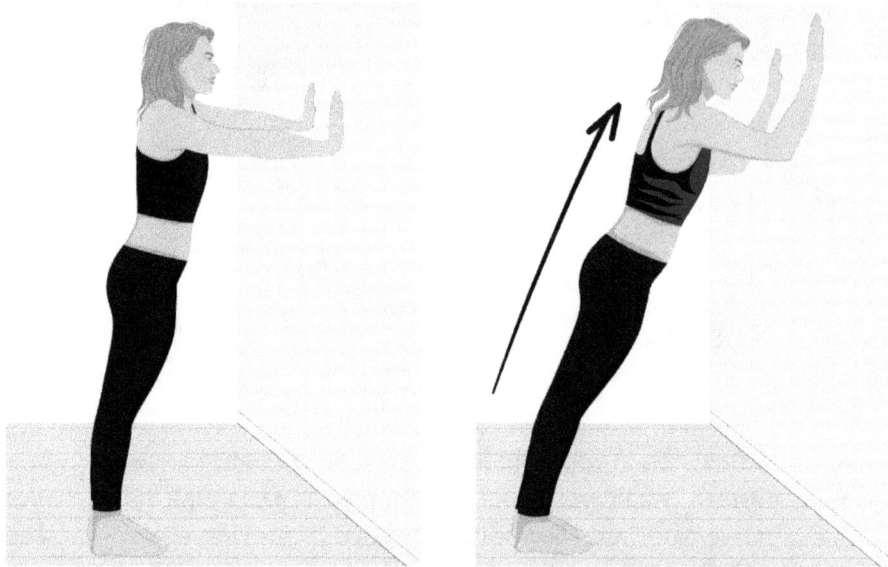

Instructions

- Stand facing a wall, about arm's length away.
- Place your palms flat against the wall at shoulder height.
- Step your feet back, leaning against the wall, and draw a straight line from your head to your heels.
- Keep your core engaged and your body straight, similar to a regular plank position.
- Hold this position for 1 minute.

Modifications

- Easier: Move your feet closer to the wall to reduce the angle and difficulty.
- Harder: Step your feet further away from the wall to increase the angle and challenge.
- Props: Place a yoga block between your hands to engage your chest muscles more.

Tips

- Keep your neck aligned with your spine, avoiding dropping or lifting your head.
- Engage your glutes and quad muscles to maintain a straight body line.
- Breathe steadily throughout the hold.
- If you feel wrist discomfort, try making fists against the wall instead of using flat palms.

Single-Leg Stretch

Single-Leg Stretches improve hamstring flexibility, strengthen the core, and enhance balance. This exercise targets multiple muscle groups simultaneously.

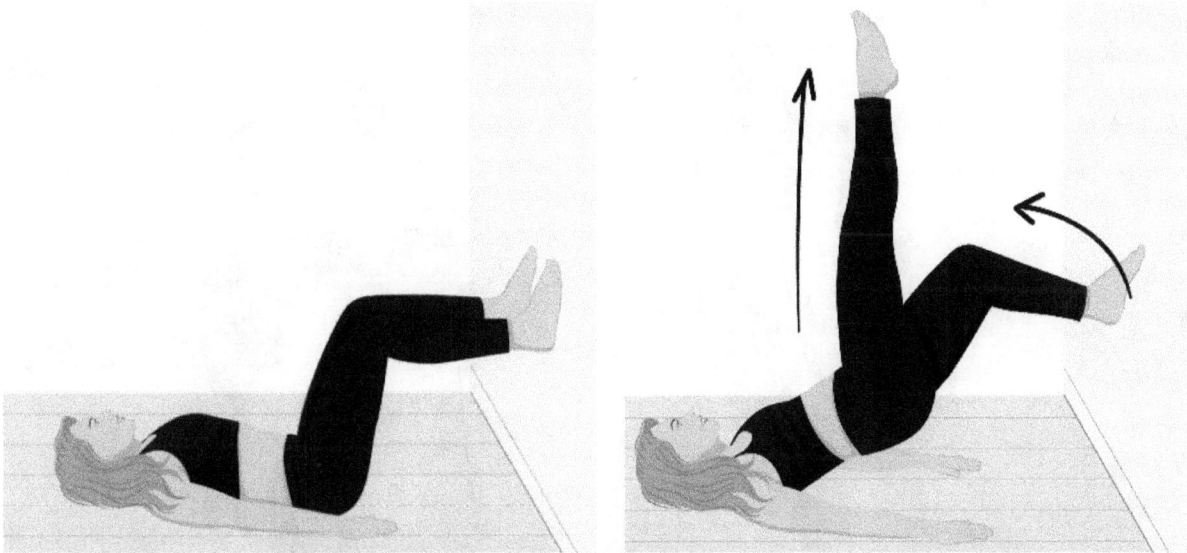

Instructions

- Lie on your back with both legs extended and resting on the wall with your knees bent.
- Lift your right leg and straighten it.
- Slowly lift your right leg toward the ceiling until you feel the stretch in your hamstring.
- If you find it challenging to keep your leg lifted unassisted, feel free to use your right hand to gently grip the back of your thigh for support.
- Hold for 30 seconds, then slowly lower the leg.
- Switch sides and repeat with the left leg for 30 seconds.

Modifications

- Easier: Bend your knee slightly if you can't keep your leg straight.
- Harder: Lift your head and shoulders off the ground to engage your core more.
- Props: Use a yoga strap around your foot to help pull your leg closer if you can't reach your ankle.

Tips

- Keep your lower back pressed into the floor throughout the movement.
- If you feel any strain in your lower back, bend your knee more or reduce the stretch.
- Breathe deeply and evenly, focusing on relaxing into the stretch.

Standing Wall Roll-Down

Standing Wall Roll-Downs improve spinal flexibility, stretch the back muscles, and promote better posture. This exercise helps decompress the spine and release tension.

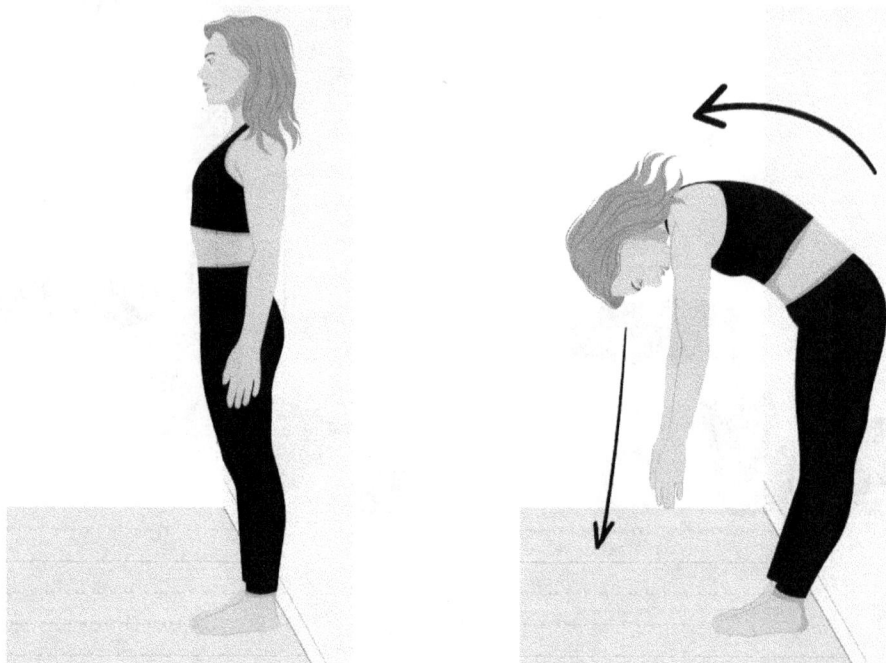

Instructions

- Stand with your back against a wall, feet hip-width apart and about 6 inches from the wall.
- Start by tucking your chin to your chest.
- Slowly roll down, peeling your spine away from the wall vertebra by vertebra.
- Continue rolling down as far as comfortable, letting your arms hang towards the floor.
- Hold the bottom position for a moment, then slowly roll back up to the starting position.
- Repeat this movement for 1 minute.

Modifications

- Easier: Don't roll down as far, focusing on the upper and mid-back areas.
- Harder: Hold the bottom position for longer before rolling back up.
- Props: Place a small cushion behind your lower back for support if needed.

Tips

- Move slowly and deliberately, focusing on each vertebra as you roll down and up.
- Breathe steadily, exhaling as you roll down and inhaling as you roll up.
- If you feel any pain or discomfort, especially in your lower back, reduce your range of motion.

Wall Push-Ups

Wall Push-Ups strengthen the chest, shoulders, and arms while being gentler on the wrists and shoulders than traditional push-ups.

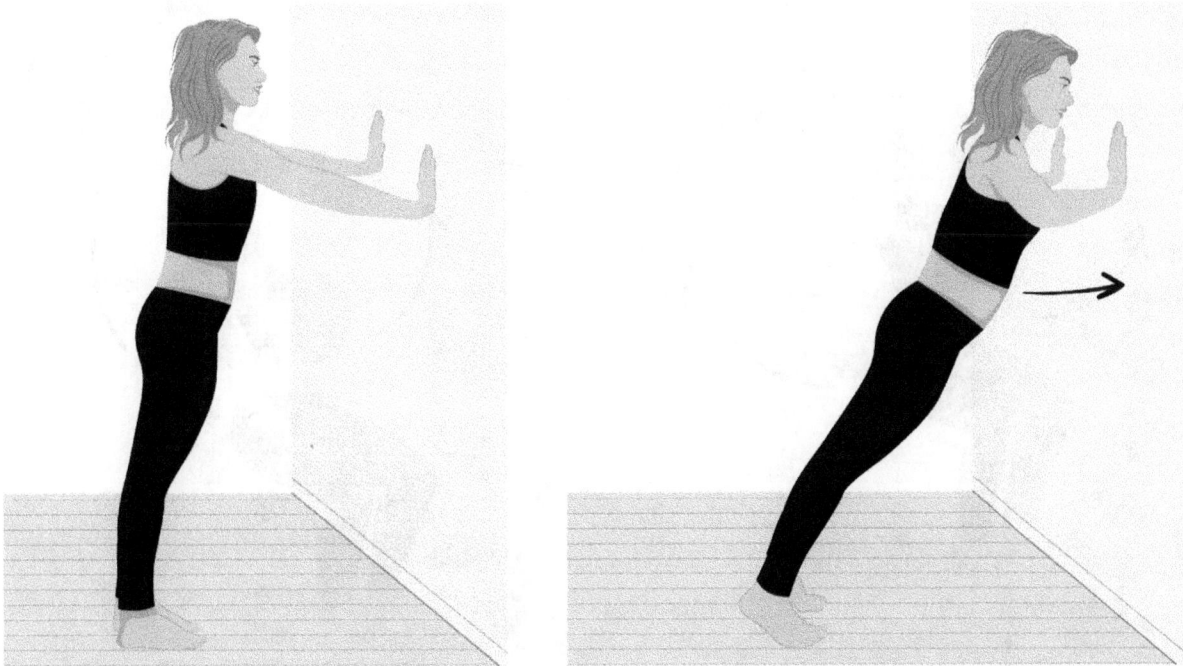

<u>Instructions</u>

- Stand arm's length from a wall; feet shoulder-width apart.
- Place your palms flat against the wall at chest height, slightly wider than shoulder width.
- Lean in towards the wall, bending your elbows to bring your chest closer to the wall.
- Push back to the starting position, straightening your arms.
- Repeat this movement for 1 minute.

<u>Modifications</u>

- Easier: Move your feet closer to the wall to reduce the angle and difficulty.
- Harder: Step further away from the wall to increase the angle and challenge.
- Props: Place a small ball between your hands to engage your chest muscles more.

<u>Tips</u>

- Keep your body in a straight line throughout the movement.
- Engage your core to maintain proper form.
- Breathe steadily, exhaling as you push away from the wall and inhaling as you lean in.

T-Press

T-presses strengthen the upper back, shoulders, and core while improving posture and shoulder stability.

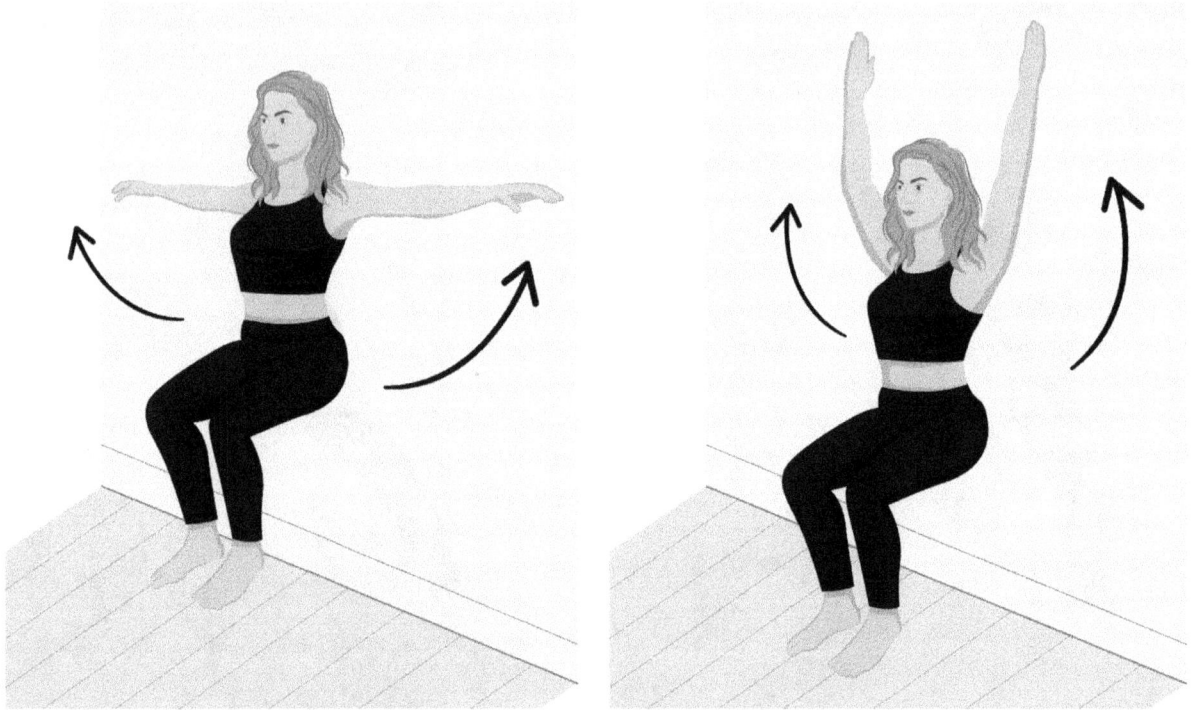

Instructions

- Stand with your back against a wall, feet hip-width apart and about 6 inches from the wall.
- Bring your arms up to form a T shape, with your arms parallel to the floor.
- Press your entire back, arms, and hands firmly against the wall.
- Maintaining this contact, slide your arms up the wall until they're straight overhead.
- Slowly lower back to the starting T position.
- Repeat this movement for 1 minute.

Modifications

- Easier: Perform the exercise with a smaller range of motion.
- Harder: Hold a light weight in each hand while performing the movement.
- Props: Use small towels under your hands to allow them to slide more easily against the wall.

Tips

- Keep your lower back pressed against the wall throughout the movement.
- Focus on squeezing your shoulder blades together as you perform the exercise.

Arm Circles

Arm Circles improve shoulder mobility, warm up the upper body, and help relieve tension in the neck and shoulders.

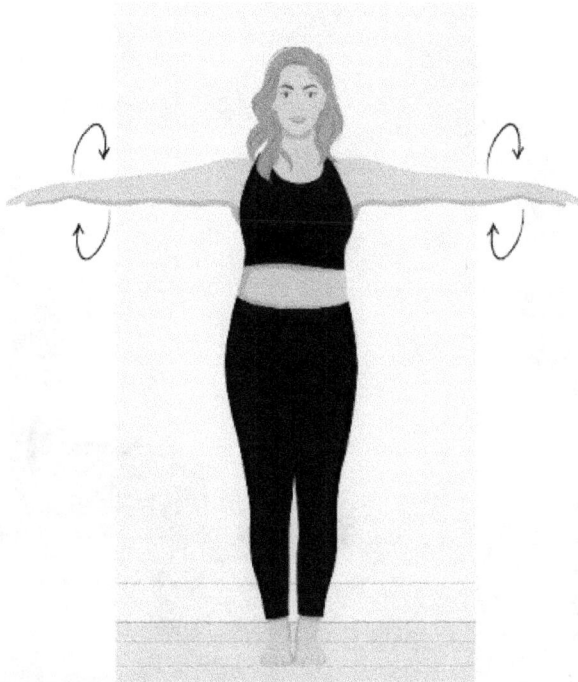

Instructions

- Stand with your feet shoulder-width apart with your back against the wall.
- Extend your arms out to the sides at shoulder height.
- Begin making small circular motions with your arms.
- Perform forward circles for 30 seconds.
- Reverse the direction and perform backward circles for 30 seconds.

Modifications

- Easier: Perform smaller circles or reduce the duration if your shoulders fatigue quickly.
- Harder: Hold light weights or water bottles while performing the circles.
- Props: Use resistance bands looped around your hands for added challenge.

Tips

- Keep your core engaged to support your lower back.
- If you experience any shoulder pain, reduce the size of your circles.
- Breathe steadily throughout the exercise.

Wall Squats

Wall Squats strengthen the quadriceps, glutes, and calves while improving lower body endurance and stability.

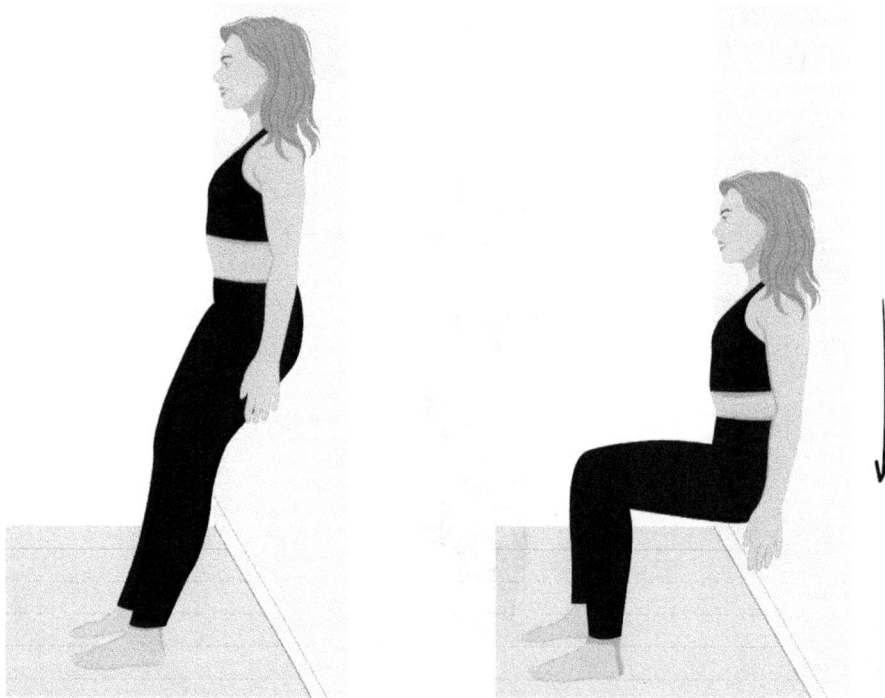

<u>Instructions</u>

- Stand with your back against a wall, feet shoulder-width apart and about 2 feet from the wall.
- Slowly slide your back down the wall until your thighs are parallel to the ground.
- Your knees should be directly above your ankles, forming a 90-degree angle.
- Slowly repeat a squat motion between the standing and squat position for 1 minute.

<u>Modifications</u>

- Easier: Don't slide down as far, maintaining a higher seated position.
- Harder: Hold light weights in your hands or extend one leg straight out in front of you while squatting, alternating legs every 15 seconds.
- Props: Place a small exercise ball between your back and the wall for added support and to help maintain proper form.

<u>Tips</u>

- Keep your core engaged throughout the hold.
- Ensure your knees don't extend past your toes.
- Focus on keeping your weight in your heels rather than your toes.

Side Leg Lifts

Side Leg Lifts target the outer thighs and hips, improving hip stability and strengthening the gluteus medius.

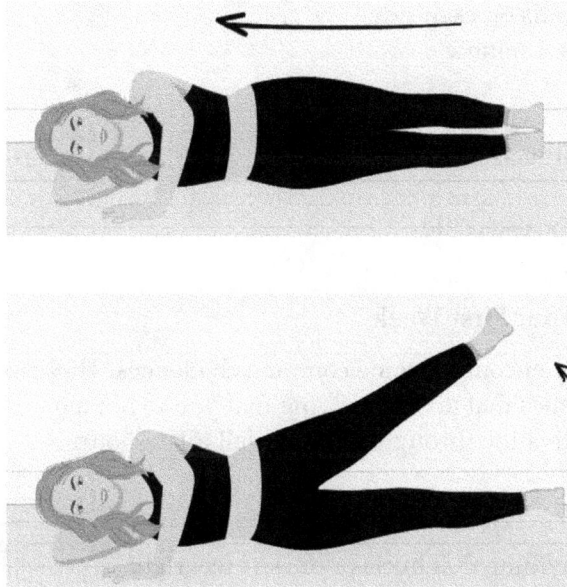

Instructions

- Lie on your right side with your legs straight and stacked on top of each other and your back against the wall for alignment.
- Support your head with your right hand, and place your left hand on the floor in front of you for balance.
- Keep your left leg straight, and slowly lift it towards the ceiling.
- Lift as high as possible while maintaining a straight leg and without rolling your hips backward.
- Lower the leg back down with control.
- Repeat for 30 seconds, then switch to the other side for 30 seconds.

Modifications

- Easier: Perform smaller leg lifts or bend your bottom leg for more stability.
- Harder: Add ankle weights or hold the leg at the top of the movement before lowering.
- Props: Use a resistance band around your ankles for added challenge.

Tips

- Keep your core engaged to maintain stability in your torso.
- Focus on lifting your leg with your hip muscles, not momentum.
- Keep your top hip stacked directly above the bottom hip throughout the movement.

Wall Pilates Routine: Day 1-4

Warm-up: 2 minutes

1. Wall Plank: 1 minute
2. Single-Leg Stretch: 30 seconds on each side
3. Standing Wall Roll-Downs: 1 minute
4. Wall Push-Ups: 1 minute
5. T-press: 1 minute
6. Arm Circles: 30 seconds on each side
7. Wall Squats: 1 minute
8. Side Leg Lifts: 30 seconds on each side

Overcoming Challenges in Your First Week

During this first week, you may encounter some common challenges. These are normal, but you must know how to overcome any issues that arise. Knowing that you're not alone and using the tips below allows you to sustain your motivation throughout your wall Pilates journey.

Listen to Your Body

- Avoid pushing through anything that hurts or doesn't feel right.
- If a routine isn't working, use the tips and modifications supplied under each exercise.
- Remember that the foundation of Pilates is the mind-body connection, so pay attention to your body and follow its lead.

Focus on Proper Alignment

- Keep your core engaged and your spine neutral throughout each exercise.
- Ensure your shoulders are down and back, your hips are level, and your feet are hip-distance apart.
- If you need to figure out if you're doing it right, double-check your form in a mirror or by recording your workout.

Breathe

- Focus on inhaling deeply through your nose and exhaling fully through your mouth, synchronizing your breath with your movements.
- If you find yourself holding your breath or getting a little lightheaded, take a break before continuing.

Adjust the Intensity

- Feel free to adjust a workout to meet your current fitness level if it feels too difficult or demanding.
- Make use of the modifications provided under each of the exercises to guide your workouts.

Day 5 to 7: Foundational Wall Pilates Exercises

Wall Plank

Wall Planks strengthen the core, improve posture, and engage the shoulders and back muscles. This exercise is excellent for building isometric strength and stability.

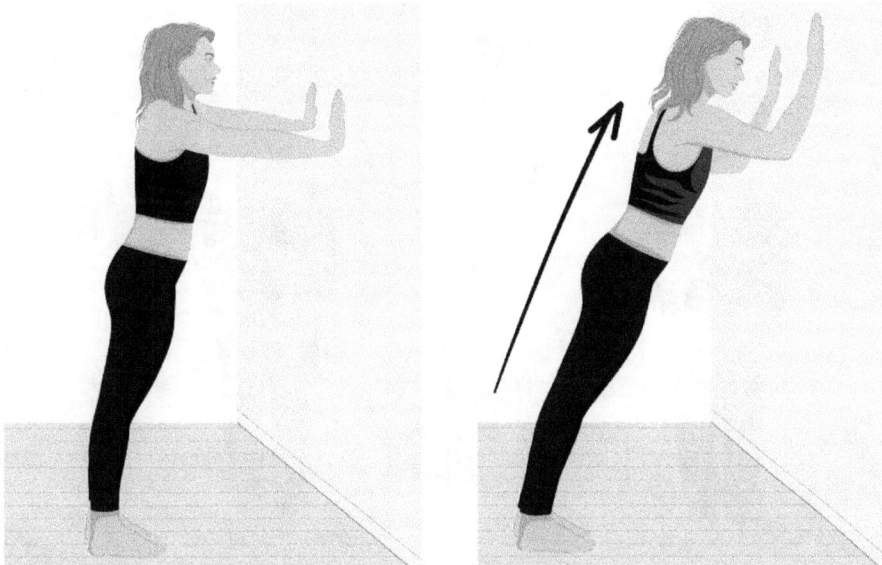

Instructions

- Stand facing a wall, about arm's length away.
- Place your palms flat against the wall at shoulder height.
- Step your feet back, leaning against the wall, and draw a straight line from your head to your heels.
- Keep your core engaged and your body straight, similar to a regular plank position.
- Hold this position for 1 minute.

Modifications

- Easier: Move your feet closer to the wall to reduce the angle and difficulty.
- Harder: Step your feet further away from the wall to increase the angle and challenge.
- Props: Place a yoga block between your hands to engage your chest muscles more.

Tips

- Keep your neck aligned with your spine, avoiding dropping or lifting your head.
- Engage your glutes and quad muscles to maintain a straight body line.
- Breathe steadily throughout the hold.
- If you feel wrist discomfort, try making fists against the wall instead of using flat palms.

Chest Fly

Chest Flies strengthen the pectoral muscles, improve chest flexibility, and engage the shoulders and arms.

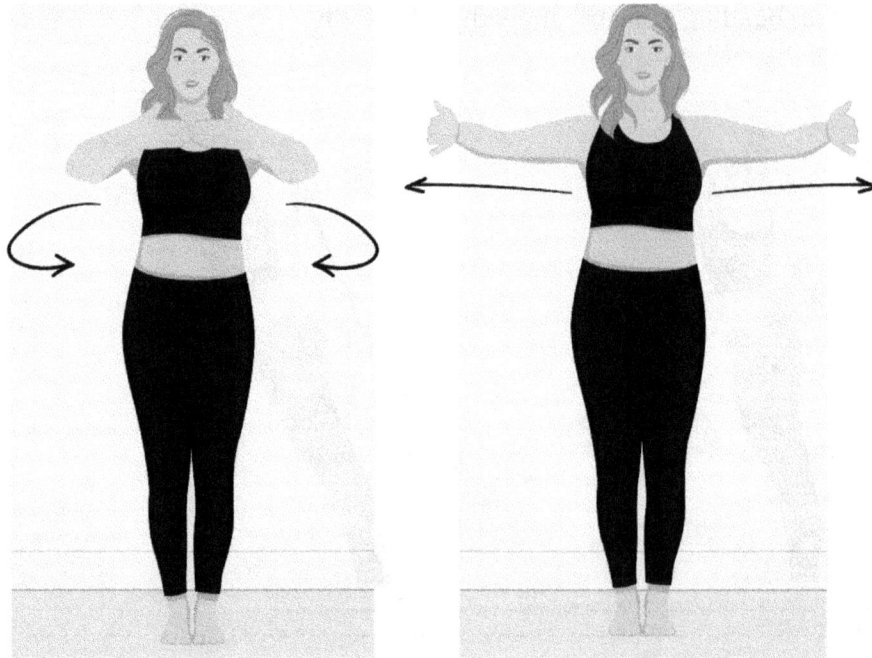

Instructions

- Stand with your back against a wall, feet about 6 inches from the base.
- Bring your arms to shoulder height, elbows bent, and press your entire back and arms against the wall.
- Bend your knees slightly to engage your thigh muscles and glutes.
- Keeping contact with the wall, bring your arms back together in front of your chest in a curved position with your left arm above the right and, the next time, your right arm above the left.
- Keep your wrists relaxed but your arms engaged.
- Repeat this movement for 1 minute.

Modifications

- Easier: Perform a smaller range of motion, not extending your arms as far.
- Harder: Hold light weights while performing the movement.

Tips

- Keep your lower back pressed against the wall throughout the movement.
- Focus on squeezing your chest muscles as you bring your arms back together.

Single-Leg Knee Crunch

Single-Leg Knee Crunches on the wall improve balance, core strength, and hip flexibility while engaging the standing leg for stability.

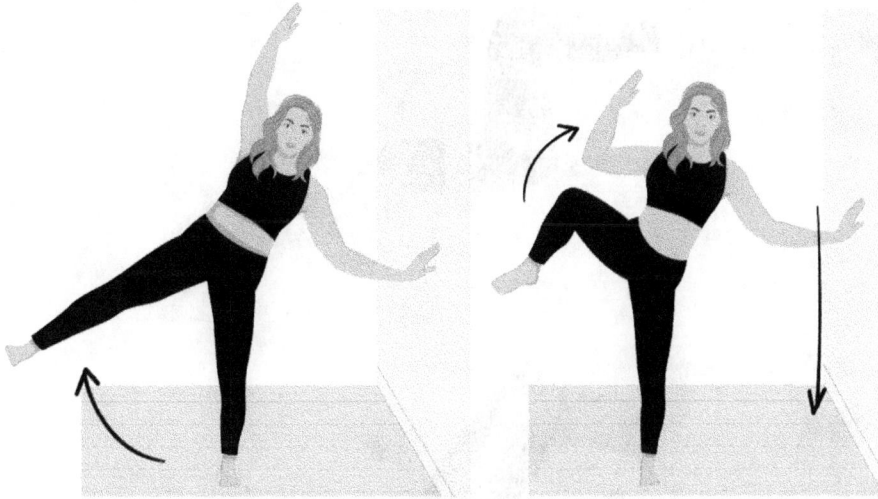

Instructions

- Stand with your right side next to the wall, feet hip-width apart, about 6 inches from the wall.
- Shift your weight onto your right leg and lift your left foot slightly off the ground.
- Raise your left arm above your head.
- Drive your left arm down toward your left leg, and as you do, lift your left knee towards your chest.
- Lower your left foot back down to the starting position.
- Repeat this movement for 30 seconds on the left side.
- Switch legs and repeat for 30 seconds on the right side.

Modifications

- Easier: Perform a smaller knee lift or maintain a higher position on the wall.
- Harder: Hold the knee-to-chest position for a count of two before lowering, or slide down the wall further (up to a 90-degree bend in the standing leg).
- Props: Hold a small exercise ball between your back and the wall for added support and to help maintain proper form.

Tips

- Keep your core engaged throughout the exercise to support your lower back.
- Maintain contact between your back and the wall during the entire movement.
- Breathe steadily, exhaling as you lift your knee and inhaling as you lower it.
- If you feel knee pain in your standing leg, reduce the depth of your slide or stop the exercise.

Wall Bridge

Wall Bridges strengthen the glutes, hamstrings, and lower back while engaging the core.

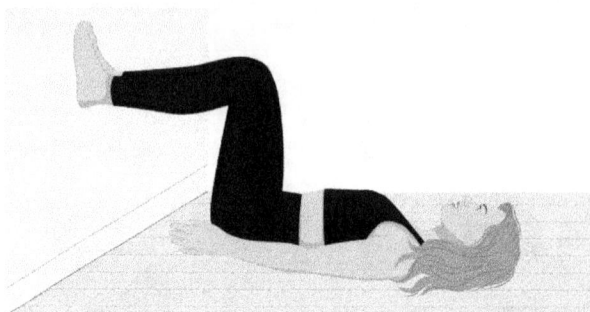

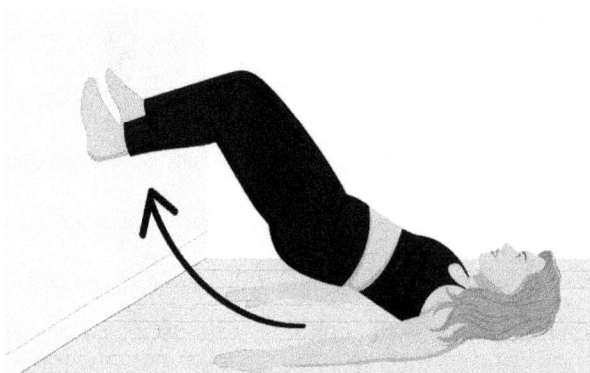

Instructions

- Lie on your back with your knees bent and feet flat against a wall, hip-width apart.
- Your arms should be at your sides, palms facing down.
- Engage your core and glutes, then slowly lift your hips off the ground until your body forms a straight line from your knees to your shoulders.
- Hold this position for 2 to 3 seconds, focusing on squeezing your glutes.
- Slowly lower your hips back to the starting position. Repeat this movement for 1 minute.

Modifications

- Easier: Perform smaller lifts, or hold the elevated position for a shorter time.
- Harder: Lift one foot off the wall at the top of the movement, holding for a few seconds before switching feet.
- Props: Place a small pillow or folded towel under your head for neck support if needed.

Tips

- Focus on pressing through your heels rather than your toes to activate your hamstrings and glutes.

Donkey Kicks

Donkey Kicks target the glutes and hamstrings, helping to strengthen the posterior chain and improve hip stability.

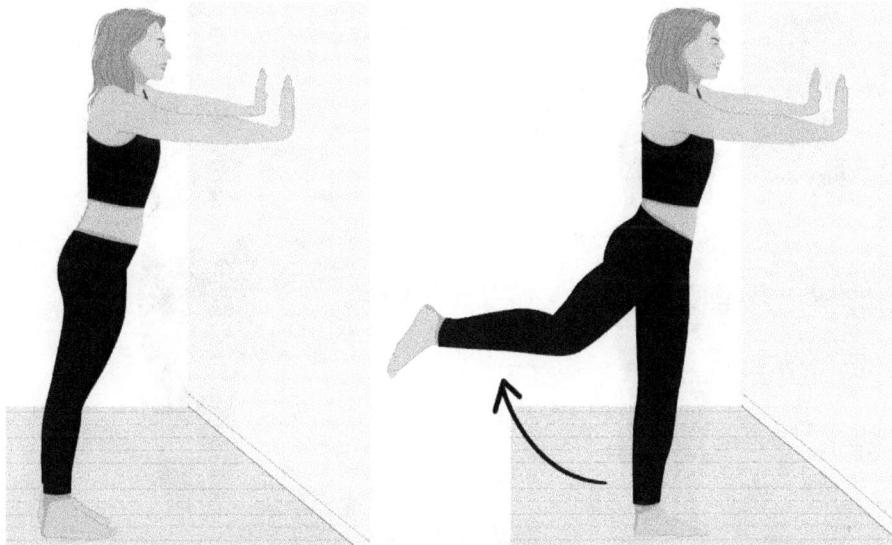

Instructions

- Begin by standing facing the wall about an arm's length away.
- Place your hands lightly on the wall at chest height for support.
- Extend your right leg straight back in a controlled motion, gently kicking while maintaining balance and stability.
- Return to the start and repeat on the other side.
- Continue these movements for 1 minute.

Modifications

- Easier: Perform smaller kicks
- Harder: Add ankle weights or hold the leg at the top of the movement for a count of two.
- Props: Use a resistance band looped around your feet

Tips

- Keep your core engaged and your back flat throughout the movement.
- Avoid arching your lower back as you lift your leg.
- Focus on squeezing your glutes at the top of the movement.

Arm Scissors

Arm Scissors strengthen the shoulders, improve upper body coordination, and engage the core for stability.

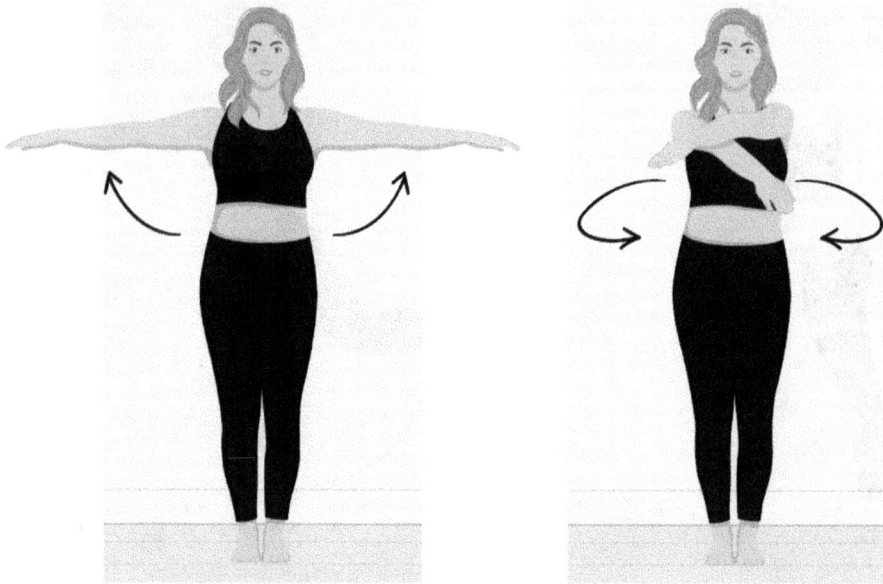

Instructions

- Stand with your feet together and your back against the wall.
- Extend your arms straight out to the sides at shoulder height.
- Keeping your arms straight, bring them in front of your body, crossing your left arm over the right.
- Open your arms back out to the sides.
- Repeat the crossing motion, this time crossing your right arm over the left.
- Continue this scissoring motion for 1 minute.

Modifications

- Easier: Perform the movement more slowly or with a smaller range of motion.
- Harder: Hold light weights or water bottles while performing the exercise.
- Props: Use resistance bands looped around your hands for added challenge.

Tips

- Keep your core engaged to maintain stability in your torso.
- Breathe steadily throughout the exercise.
- If you feel any shoulder discomfort, reduce the range of motion or speed.

Side Leg Lifts

Side Leg Lifts target the outer thighs and hips, improving hip stability and strengthening the gluteus medius.

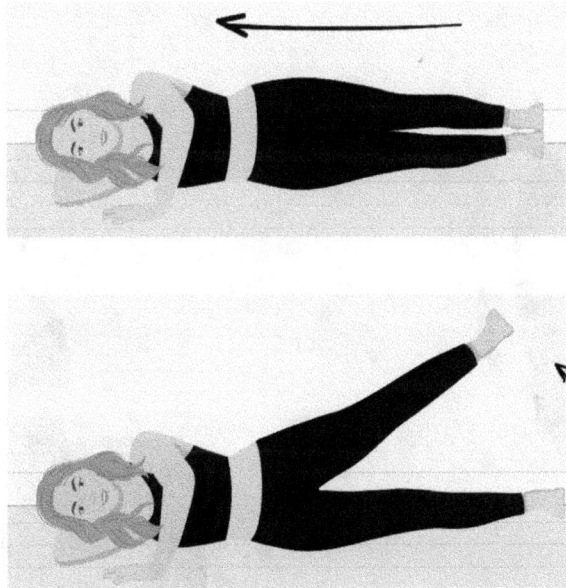

<u>Instructions</u>

- Lie on your right side with your legs straight and stacked on top of each other.
- Support your head with your right hand, and place your left hand on the floor in front of you for balance.
- Keeping your left leg straight, slowly lift it towards the ceiling.
- Lift as high as possible while maintaining a straight leg and without rolling your hips backward.
- Lower the leg back down with control.
- Repeat for 30 seconds, then switch to the other side for 30 seconds.

<u>Modifications</u>

- Easier: Perform smaller leg lifts or bend your bottom leg for more stability.
- Harder: Add ankle weights or hold the leg at the top of the movement before lowering.
- Props: Use a resistance band around your ankles for added challenge.

<u>Tips</u>

- Keep your core engaged to maintain stability in your torso.
- Focus on lifting your leg with your hip muscles, not momentum.
- Keep your top hip stacked directly above the bottom hip throughout the movement.

Wall Squats

Wall Squats strengthen the quadriceps, glutes, and calves while improving lower body endurance and stability.

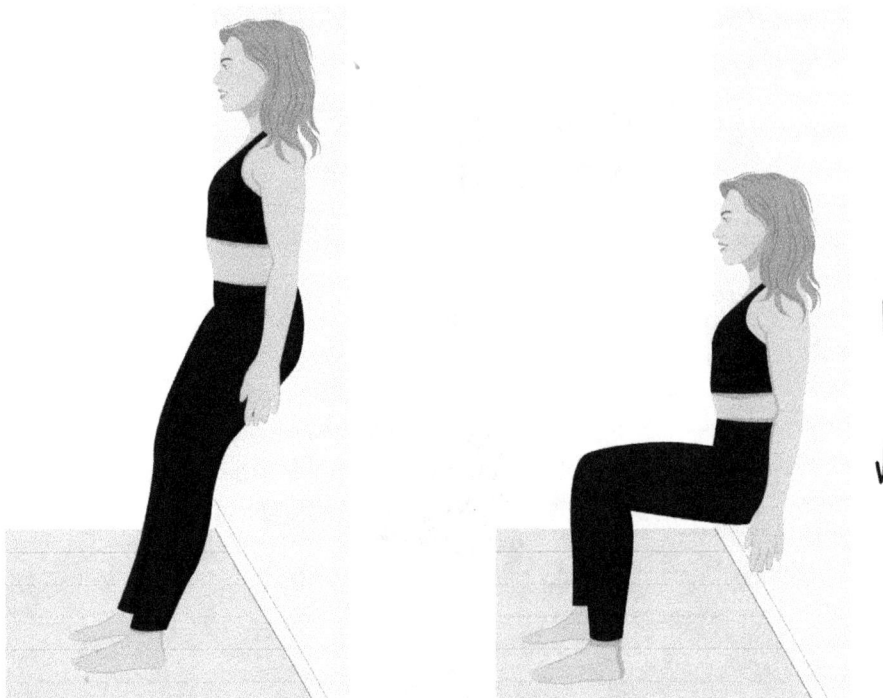

<u>Instructions</u>

- Stand with your back against a wall, feet shoulder-width apart and about 2 feet from the wall.
- Slowly slide your back down the wall until your thighs parallel the ground.
- Your knees should be directly above your ankles, forming a 90-degree angle.
- Repeat a squat motion between the standing and squat positions for 1 minute.

<u>Modifications</u>

- Easier: Don't slide down as far, maintaining a higher seated position.
- Harder: Hold light weights in your hands or extend one leg straight out in front of you while squatting, alternating legs every 15 seconds.
- Props: Place a small exercise ball between your back and the wall for added support and to help maintain proper form.

<u>Tips</u>

- Keep your core engaged throughout the hold.
- Ensure your knees don't extend past your toes.
- Focus on keeping your weight in your heels rather than your toes.

Wall Pilates Routine: Day 5-7

Warm-up: 2 minutes

1. Wall Plank: 1 minute
2. Chest Fly: 1 minute
3. Single-leg knee Crunch: 30 seconds on each side
4. Wall Bridge: 1 minute
5. Donkey Kicks: 1 minute
6. Arm Scissors: 1 minute
7. Side Leg Lifts: 30 seconds on each side
8. Wall Squats: 1 minute

Completing each of the exercises provided to you this week and using the modifications available to you will set you up for the coming week. Remember to nourish your body throughout this week and ensure that you are adequately hydrated to be strong and healthy for week 2.

CHAPTER 5
WEEK 2—EXPANDING ON YOUR WALL PILATES WORKOUTS

*T*his week, you will build on the foundational exercises you have been practicing. This week focuses on building strength and stability to support you in the later weeks of this challenge.

Challenging yourself can feel daunting, particularly if you're new to wall Pilates or exercise in general. The exercises during this week should meet you where you are in your wall Pilates journey; however, modifications have been provided.

Progression from Foundational Exercises to More Challenging Ones

To avoid plateauing, it's important to change things up and incorporate new movements that continue to challenge you. This strategic progression ensures you do not experience too much downtime when it comes to muscle pain while still encouraging your body to become stronger. In addition, during this week, as you take on more challenging movements, you should begin to see or feel tangible results.

During this week, you can expect to

- use some of the foundational exercises from week 1.
- gradually implement new movements that challenge different muscle groups or more deeply engage muscles that have already been worked on.
- incorporate props as your body adjusts to slightly more intense exercises,

As you progress through this week, listen to your body and work within your limitations. Instead of aiming to complete a large number of reps in the provided time, focus on form and alignment and use the modifications provided.

Day 8 to 11: Wall Pilates Exercises

T-Press

T-presses strengthen the upper back, shoulders, and core while improving posture and stability.

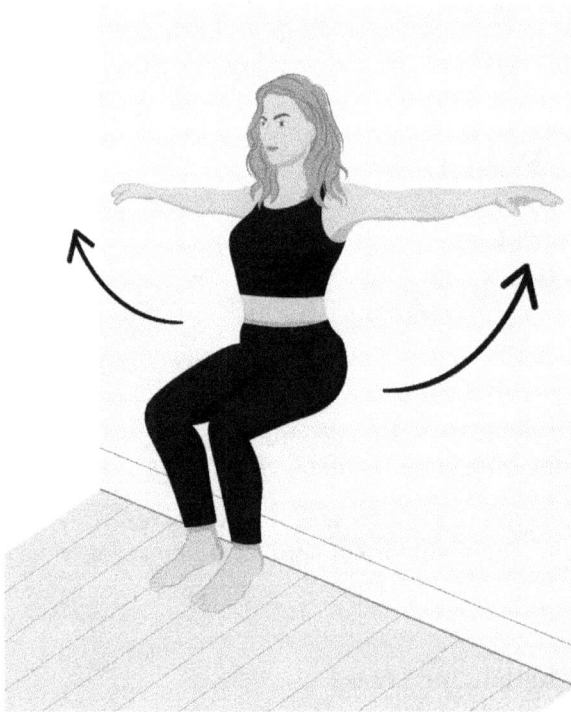

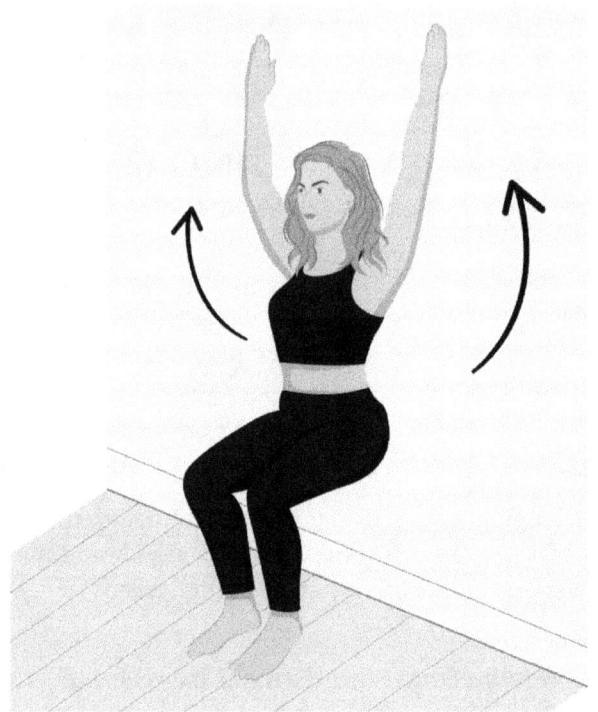

Instructions

- Stand with your back against a wall, feet hip-width apart and about 6 inches from the wall.
- Bring your arms up to form a T shape, with your arms parallel to the floor.
- Press your entire back, arms, and hands firmly against the wall.
- Maintaining this contact, slide your arms up the wall until they're straight overhead.
- Slowly lower back to the starting T position. Repeat this movement for 1 minute.

Modifications

- Easier: Perform the exercise with a smaller range of motion.
- Harder: Hold a light weight in each hand while performing the movement.
- Props: Use small towels under your hands to allow them to slide more easily against the wall.

Tips

- Keep your lower back pressed against the wall throughout the movement.
- Focus on squeezing your shoulder blades together as you perform the exercise.

Arm Scissors

Arm Scissors strengthen the shoulders, improve upper body coordination, and engage the core for stability.

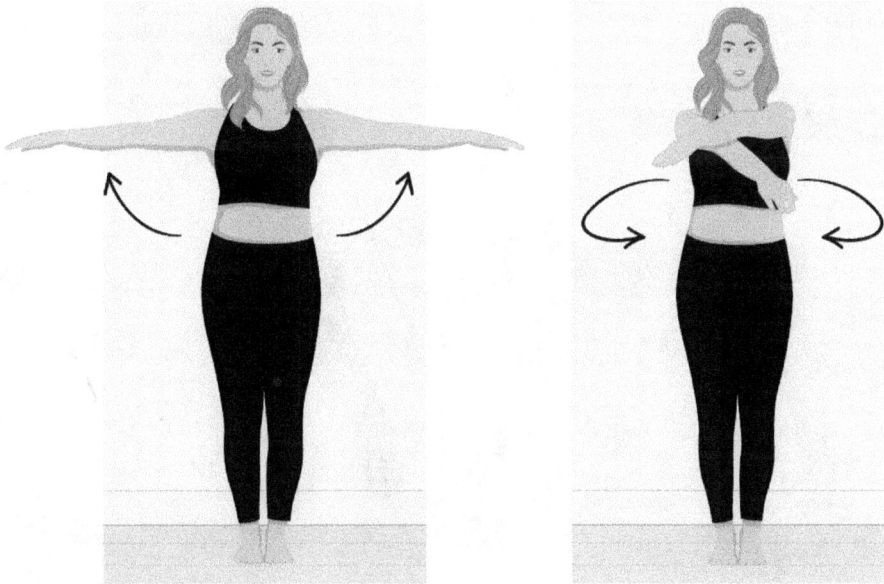

Instructions

- Stand with your feet together and your back against the wall.
- Extend your arms straight out to the sides at shoulder height.
- Keep your arms straight, bring them in front of your body, and cross your left arm over the right.
- Open your arms back out to the sides.
- Repeat the crossing motion, this time crossing your right arm over the left.
- Continue this scissoring motion for 1 minute.

Modifications

- Easier: Perform the movement more slowly or with a smaller range of motion.
- Harder: Hold light weights or water bottles while performing the exercise.
- Props: Use resistance bands looped around your hands for added challenge.

Tips

- Keep your core engaged to maintain stability in your torso.
- Breathe steadily throughout the exercise.
- If you feel any shoulder discomfort, reduce the range of motion or speed.

Wall Plank

Wall Planks strengthen the core, improve posture, and engage the shoulders and back muscles. This exercise is excellent for building isometric strength and stability.

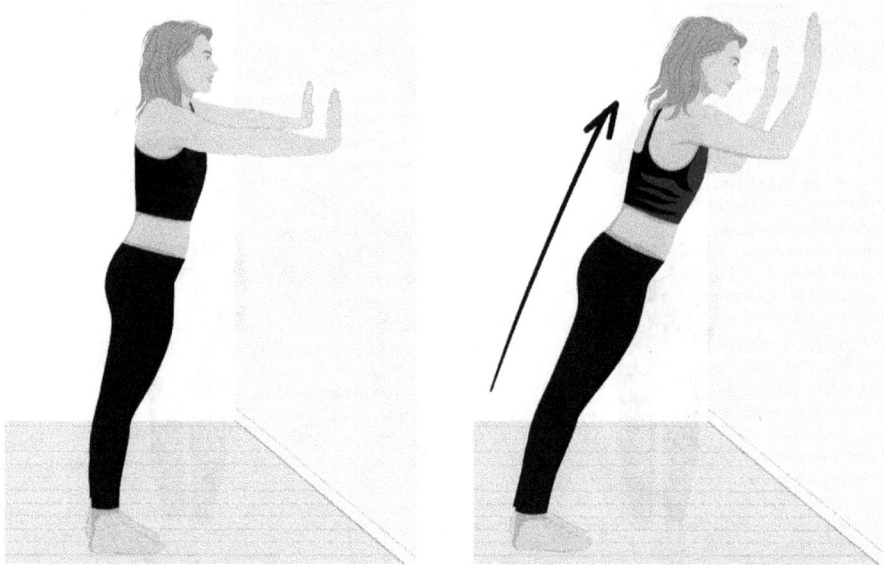

<u>Instructions</u>

- Stand facing a wall, about arm's length away.
- Place your palms flat against the wall at shoulder height.
- Step your feet back, leaning against the wall, and draw a straight line from your head to your heels.
- Keep your core engaged and your body straight, similar to a regular plank position.
- Hold this position for 1 minute.

<u>Modifications</u>

- Easier: Move your feet closer to the wall to reduce the angle and difficulty.
- Harder: Step your feet further away from the wall to increase the angle and challenge.
- Props: Place a yoga block between your hands to engage your chest muscles more.

<u>Tips</u>

- Keep your neck aligned with your spine, avoiding dropping or lifting your head.
- Engage your glutes and quad muscles to maintain a straight body line.
- Breathe steadily throughout the hold.
- If you feel wrist discomfort, try making fists against the wall instead of using flat palms.

Chest Fly

Chest Flies strengthen the pectoral muscles, improve chest flexibility, and engage the shoulders and arms.

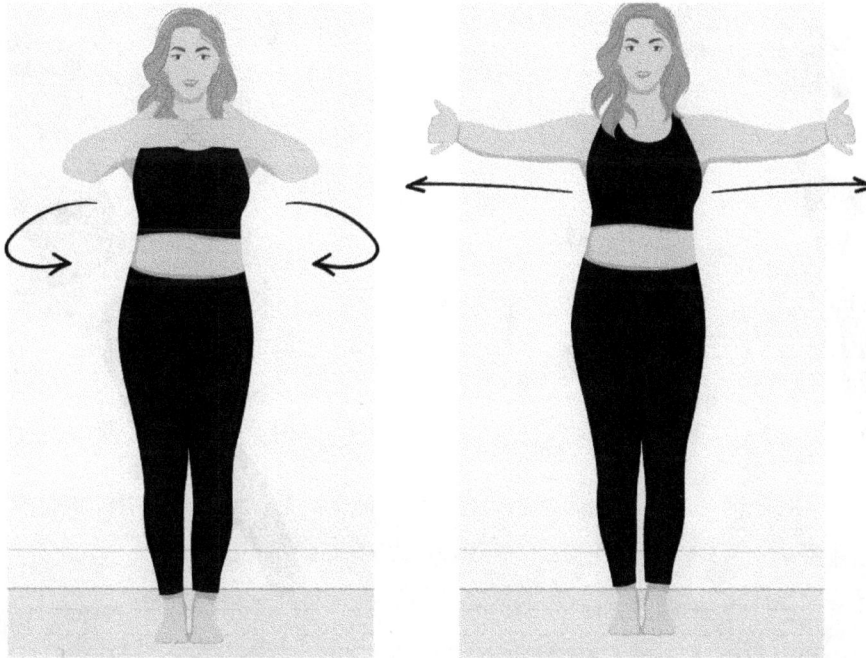

Instructions

- Stand with your back against a wall, feet about 6 inches from the base.
- Bring your arms to shoulder height, elbows bent, and press your entire back and arms against the wall.
- Bend your knees slightly to engage your thigh muscles and glutes.
- Keeping contact with the wall, bring your arms back together in front of your chest in a curved position with your left arm above the right and, the next time, your right arm above the left.
- Keep your wrists relaxed but your arms engaged.
- Repeat this movement for 1 minute.

Modifications

- Easier: Perform a smaller range of motion, not extending your arms as far.
- Harder: Hold light weights while performing the movement.

Tips

- Keep your lower back pressed against the wall throughout the movement.
- Focus on squeezing your chest muscles as you bring your arms back together.

Wall Push-Ups

Wall Push-Ups strengthen the chest, shoulders, and arms while being gentler on the wrists and shoulders than traditional push-ups.

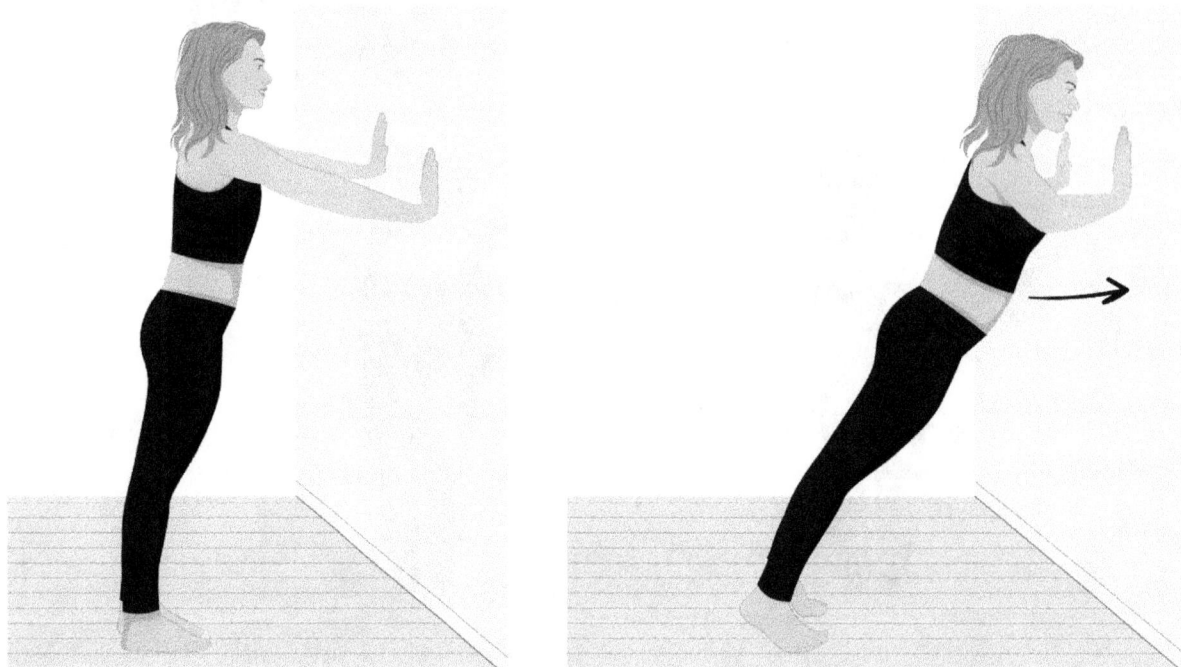

Instructions

- Stand arm's length from a wall; feet shoulder-width apart.
- Place your palms flat against the wall at chest height, slightly wider than shoulder width.
- Lean in towards the wall, bending your elbows to bring your chest closer to the wall.
- Push back to the starting position, straightening your arms.
- Repeat this movement for 1 minute.

Modifications

- Easier: Move your feet closer to the wall to reduce the angle and difficulty.
- Harder: Step further away from the wall to increase the angle and challenge.
- Props: Place a small ball between your hands to engage your chest muscles more.

Tips

- Keep your body in a straight line throughout the movement.
- Engage your core to maintain proper form.
- Breathe steadily, exhaling as you push away from the wall and inhaling as you lean in.

Alternate Leg Flexion

Alternate Leg Flexion improves hip flexibility, strengthens the core, and enhances lower-body coordination.

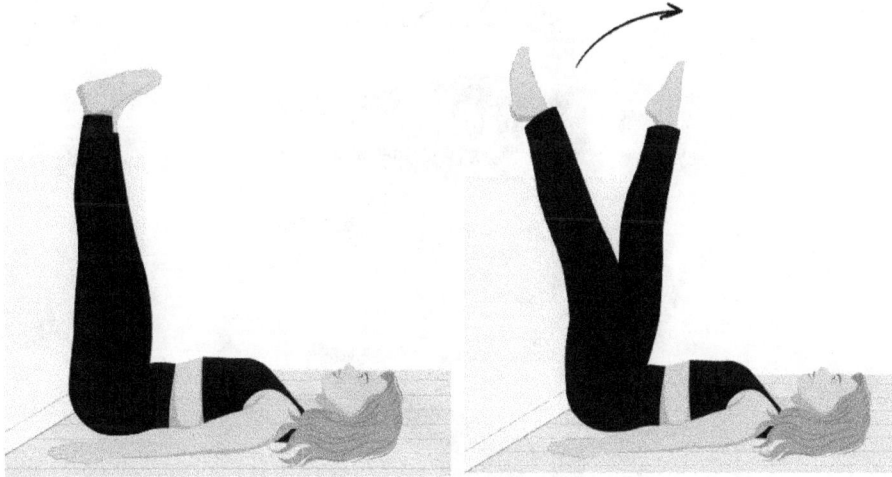

Instructions

- Lie on your back on the floor with your buttocks close to a wall, about 6 inches away.
- Extend both legs up the wall, bending your knees.
- Your body should form an inverted L shape, with your back on the floor and legs up the wall.
- Keep your upper back, shoulders, and head in contact with the floor throughout the exercise.
- Place your arms at your sides, palms down, for stability.
- Lift your right foot off the wall, moving your thigh towards your chest.
- Hold for 2-3 seconds, then slowly move your right foot back to the wall.
- Lift your left foot in the same manner.
- Continue alternating legs for 1 minute.

Modifications

- Easier: Make smaller movements or slightly bend your knee.
- Harder: Hold each leg lift for 5 seconds before switching.
- Props: Use a small pillow under your lower back if you feel pain or discomfort.

Tips

- Keep your core engaged throughout the exercise to support your lower back.
- Maintain contact between your upper back and the floor during the entire movement.

Side Leg Lifts

Side Leg Lifts target the outer thighs and hips, improving hip stability and strengthening the gluteus medius.

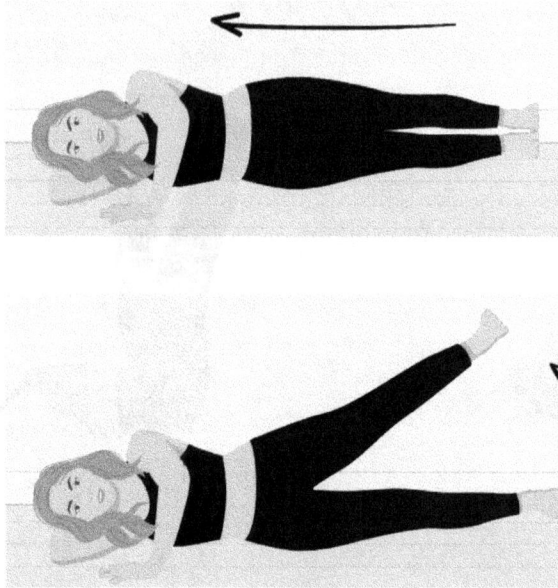

Instructions

- Lie on your right side with your legs straight and stacked on top of each other.
- Support your head with your right hand, and place your left hand on the floor in front of you for balance.
- Keep your left leg straight, and slowly lift it towards the ceiling.
- Lift as high as possible while maintaining a straight leg and without rolling your hips backward.
- Lower the leg back down with control.
- Repeat for 30 seconds, then switch to the other side for 30 seconds.

Modifications

- Easier: Perform smaller leg lifts or bend your bottom leg for more stability.
- Harder: Add ankle weights or hold the leg at the top of the movement before lowering.
- Props: Use a resistance band around your ankles for added challenge.

Tips

- Keep your core engaged to maintain stability in your torso.
- Focus on lifting your leg with your hip muscles, not momentum.
- Keep your top hip stacked directly above the bottom hip throughout the movement.

Wall Mountain Climbers

Wall Mountain Climbers provide a low-impact cardiovascular workout while engaging the core, hip flexors, and legs.

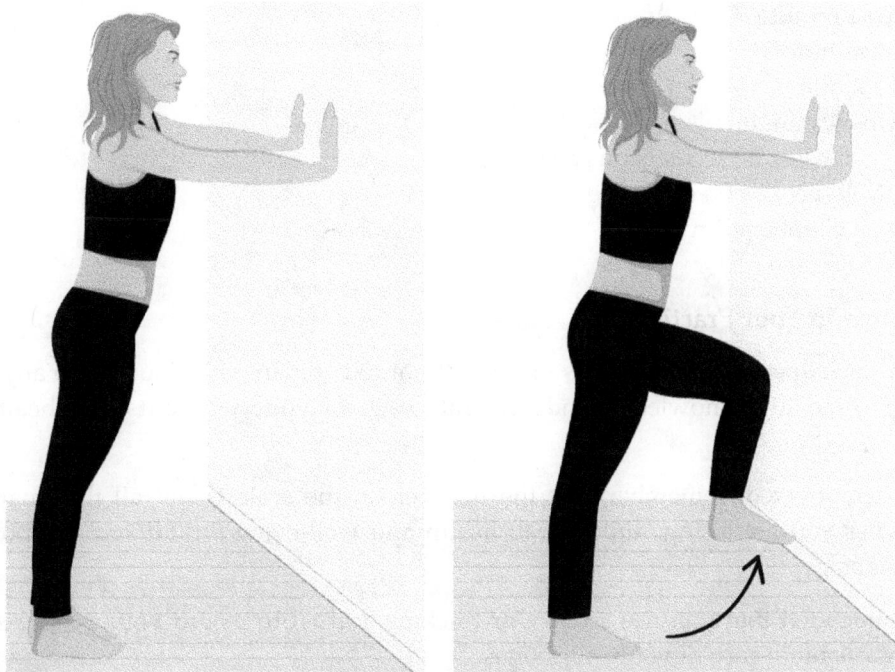

Instructions

- Start in a wall plank position, hands against the wall at shoulder height, body in a straight line.
- Bring your right knee to your chest, then return it to the starting position.
- Immediately bring your left knee up towards your chest, then return it.
- Continue alternating legs in a running motion.
- Perform this exercise for 1 minute.

Modifications

- Easier: Perform the movement more slowly or bring your knees up to a lower height.
- Harder: Increase the speed of the movement, raise your legs higher, or step your feet further away from the wall.
- Props: Place sliders or small towels under your feet to reduce friction with the floor.

Tips

- Keep your core engaged throughout the exercise to maintain a straight body line.
- Breathe steadily, finding a rhythm with your movements.

Wall Pilates Routine: Day 8-11

Warm-up: 2 minutes

1. T-Press: 1 minute
2. Arm Scissors: 1 minute
3. Wall Plank: 1 minute
4. Chest Fly: 1 minute
5. Wall Push-Ups: 1 minute
6. Alternate Leg Flexion: 30 seconds on each side
7. Side Leg Lift: 30 seconds on each side
8. Wall Mountain Climbers: 1 minute

Staying Motivated in Your Practice

Everyone's path to wellness is different. It's important not to compare your journey to anyone else's. Instead, take the time to acknowledge and celebrate each of your workouts and healthy eating milestones.

If you become demotivated, remember that the number on the scale is not all that matters. Your strength, the inches you are losing, and overall health and well-being are far more important than weight loss at this stage.

It's highly recommended that you use a diary or tracking journal to record your progress, set your fitness goals, and celebrate each of your milestones.

Keep an eye out for your gift, which will help you keep track of everything during your 4-week program.

Day 12 to 14: Wall Pilates Exercises

Forward Lunge

Forward Wall Lunges strengthen the quadriceps, hamstrings, and glutes while improving balance and hip mobility.

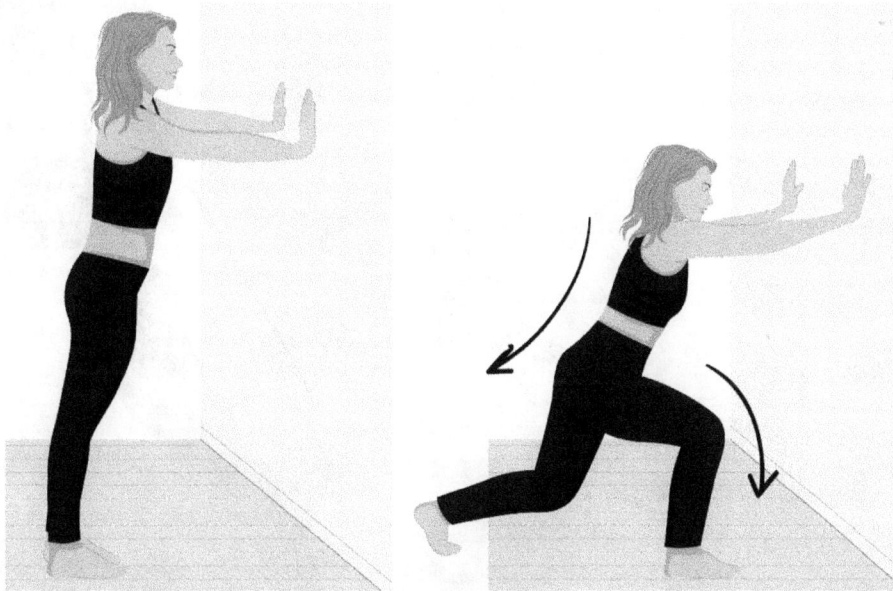

<u>Instructions</u>

- Stand facing the wall, about arm's length away.
- Place your palms flat against the wall at chest height for support.
- Take a large step forward with your right foot, keeping your left foot in place.
- Bend both knees to lower your body, keeping your front knee aligned over your ankle.
- Lower yourself until your back knee is a few inches from the ground or as far as comfortable.
- Push through your front heel to return to the starting position.
- Repeat with the left leg stepping forward.
- Continue alternating legs for 1 minute.

<u>Modifications</u>

- Easier: Start closer to the wall, take a smaller step forward, and don't lower as deeply.
- Harder: Hold the lunge position for 2-3 seconds before pushing back up, or add a knee lift with the front leg before stepping forward.
- Props: Hold light dumbbells at your sides for added resistance.

<u>Tips</u>

- Keep your chest up and shoulders back, avoiding leaning into the wall.

Shoulder Press

The shoulder press is very similar to push-ups, but by slightly changing your hand position, you target the shoulder muscles instead of the chest.

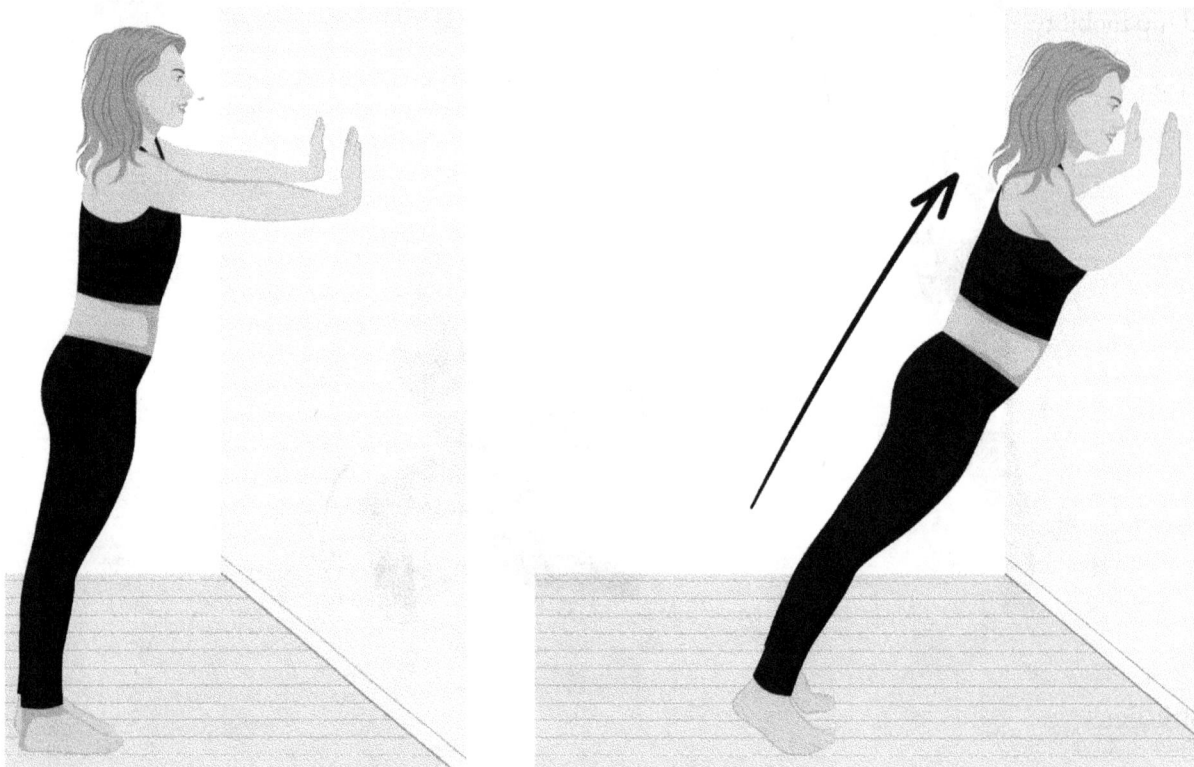

- Stand facing the wall, about an arm's length away, with your feet hip-width apart.
- Place your hands on the wall at shoulder height, fingers pointing up.
- Bend your elbows to lower your chest towards the wall, keeping your core engaged and your body straight.
- Press through your hands to straighten your arms, returning to the starting position.
- Repeat for 1 minute.

Modifications

- Easier: Step closer to the wall.
- Harder: Step a bit further away from the wall.

Tips

- Keep your core engaged throughout the movement.
- Breathe steadily: inhale as you lower, exhale as you push up.
- Keep your body in a straight line from hands to hips.

Wall Squats

Wall Squats strengthen the quadriceps, glutes, and calves while improving lower body endurance and stability.

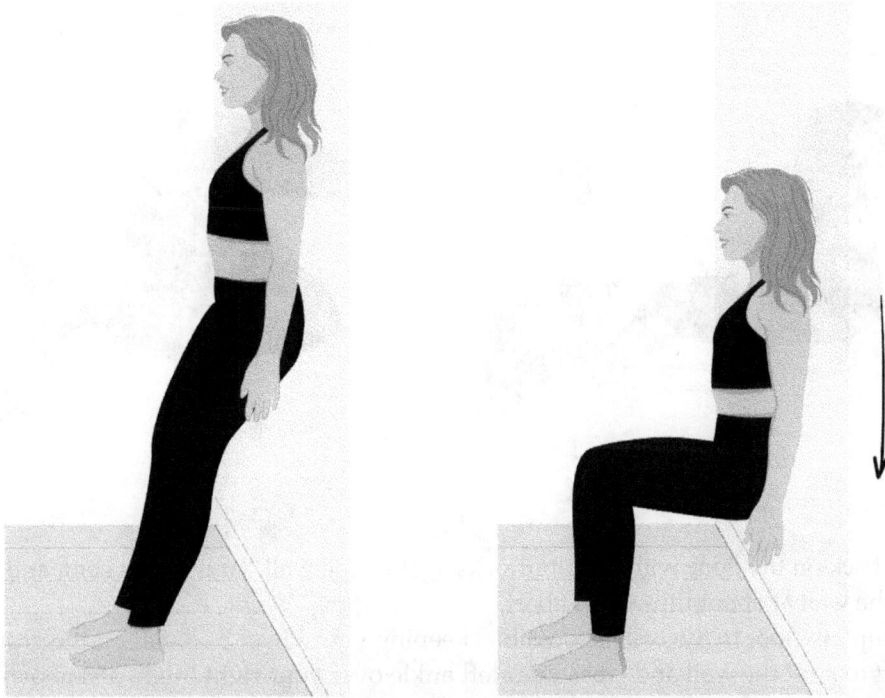

Instructions

- Stand with your back against a wall, feet shoulder-width apart and about 2 feet from the wall.
- Slowly slide your back down the wall until your thighs parallel the ground.
- Your knees should be directly above your ankles, forming a 90-degree angle.
- Repeat a squat motion between the standing and squat positions for 1 minute.

Modifications

- Easier: Don't slide down as far, maintaining a higher seated position.
- Harder: Hold light weights in your hands or extend one leg straight out in front of you while squatting, alternating legs every 15 seconds.
- Props: Place a small exercise ball between your back and the wall for added support and to help maintain proper form.

Tips

- Keep your core engaged throughout the hold.
- Ensure your knees don't extend past your toes.
- Focus on keeping your weight in your heels rather than your toes.

Wall Figure Four

Wall Figure Four stretches the glutes, piriformis, and outer hip muscles while improving balance and hip mobility.

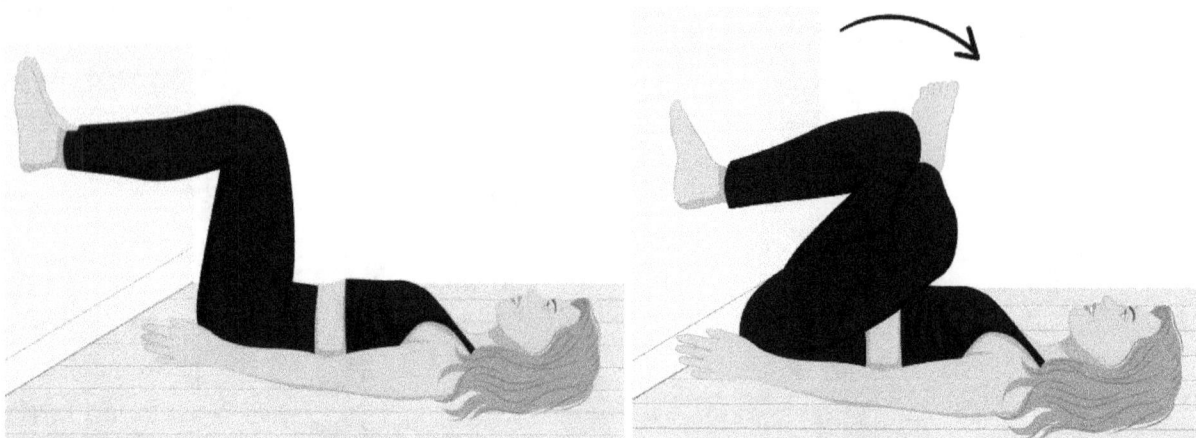

Instructions

- Lie on your back on the floor with your buttocks against the wall, your knees bent, and your feet flat on the wall at about hip-width apart.
- Scoot your hips as close to the wall as possible, keeping your lower back flat on the ground.
- Lift your left foot off the wall and cross your left ankle over your right thigh, just above the knee.
- Your left leg should form a "4" shape against the wall.
- Gently press your left knee away from your body to deepen the stretch.
- Hold this position for 30 seconds.
- Uncross your legs and return both feet to the wall.
- Repeat on the other side, crossing your right ankle over your left thigh for 30 seconds.

Modifications

- Easier: Position yourself further from the wall to decrease the intensity of the stretch.
- Harder: Gently push your foot into the wall to increase the stretch in your opposite hip.
- Props: Place a folded towel or small pillow under your head for neck support if needed.

Tips

- Keep your lower back pressed into the floor throughout the exercise.
- If the stretch is too intense, move your hips slightly away from the wall.

Wall Bridge

Wall Bridges strengthen the glutes, hamstrings, and lower back while engaging the core.

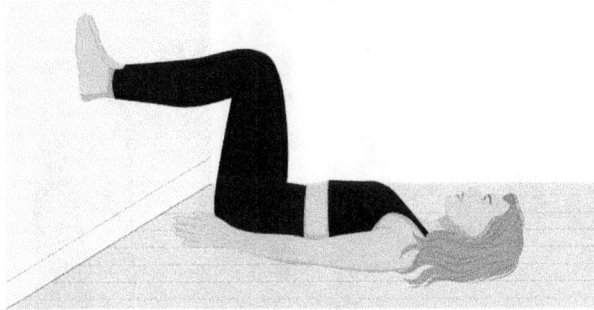

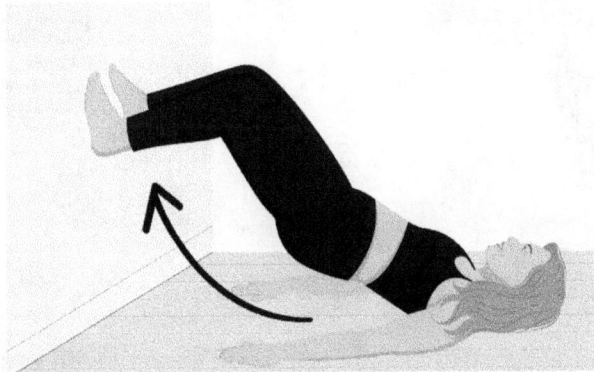

Instructions

- Lie on your back with your knees bent and feet flat against a wall, hip-width apart.
- Your arms should be at your sides, palms facing down.
- Engage your core and glutes, then slowly lift your hips off the ground until your body forms a straight line from your knees to your shoulders.
- Hold this position for 2 to 3 seconds, focusing on squeezing your glutes.
- Slowly lower your hips back to the starting position. Repeat this movement for 1 minute.

Modifications

- Easier: Perform smaller lifts, or hold the elevated position for a shorter time.
- Harder: Lift one foot off the wall at the top of the movement, holding for a few seconds before switching feet.
- Props: Place a small pillow or folded towel under your head for neck support if needed.

Tips

- Focus on pressing through your heels rather than your toes to activate your hamstrings and glutes.

Single-Leg Stretch

Single-Leg Stretches improve hamstring flexibility, strengthen the core, and enhance balance. This exercise targets multiple muscle groups simultaneously.

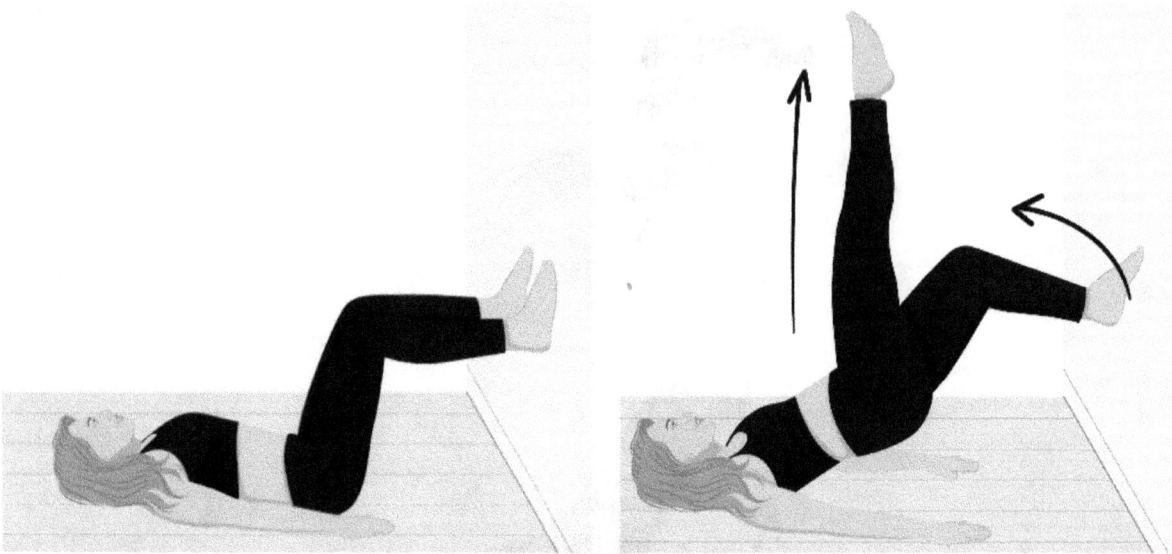

Instructions

- Lie on your back with both legs extended and resting on the wall with your knees bent.
- Lift your right leg and straighten it.
- Slowly lift your right leg toward the ceiling until you feel the stretch in your hamstring.
- If you find it challenging to keep your leg lifted unassisted, feel free to use your right hand to grip the back of your thigh for support gently.
- Hold for 30 seconds, then slowly lower the leg.
- Switch sides and repeat with the left leg for 30 seconds.

Modifications

- Easier: Bend your knee slightly if you can't keep your leg straight.
- Harder: Lift your head and shoulders off the ground to engage your core more.
- Props: Use a yoga strap around your foot to help pull your leg closer if you can't reach your ankle.

Tips

- Keep your lower back pressed into the floor throughout the movement.
- If you feel any strain in your lower back, bend your knee more or reduce the stretch.
- Breathe deeply and evenly, focusing on relaxing into the stretch.

Wall Marches

Wall Marches in this position strengthen the core, particularly the lower abdominals, while engaging the hip flexors and improving overall body control.

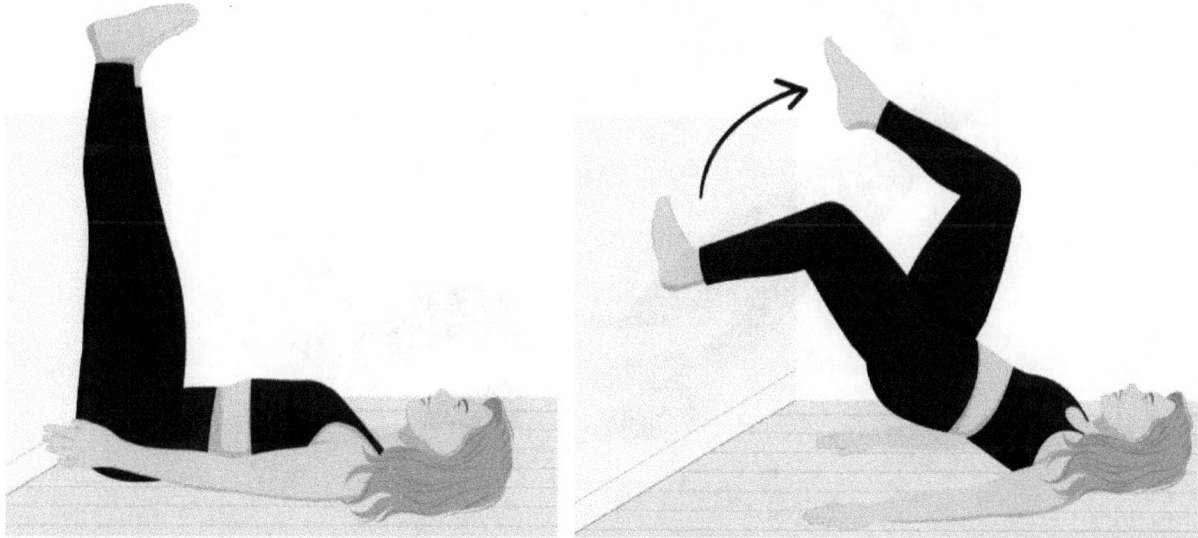

<u>Instructions</u>

- Lie on your back with your hips close to the wall.
- Extend your legs up the wall, keeping them straight so your body forms an "L" shape.
- Place your arms at your sides, palms down, for stability.
- Engage your core and press your lower back into the floor.
- Lift your right foot about 6 to 12 inches off the wall, bending at the hip and knee.
- Lower your right foot back to the wall.
- Immediately lift your left foot in the same manner.
- Continue alternating legs in a marching motion for 1 minute.

<u>Modifications</u>

- Easier: Perform smaller lifts, raising your feet only a few inches off the wall.
- Harder: Hold each leg lift for 2-3 seconds before switching.
- Props: Place a small pillow under your head for neck support if needed.

<u>Tips</u>

- Keep your lower back pressed firmly against the floor throughout the exercise.
- Engage your core muscles to maintain stability and protect your lower back.
- Breathe steadily, exhaling as you lift your foot and inhaling as you lower it.
- If you feel any strain in your lower back, reduce the range of motion or stop the exercise.
- Focus on controlled movements rather than speed.

100s

Wall 100s intensely engage the core muscles, particularly the lower abdominals, while using the wall for leg support.

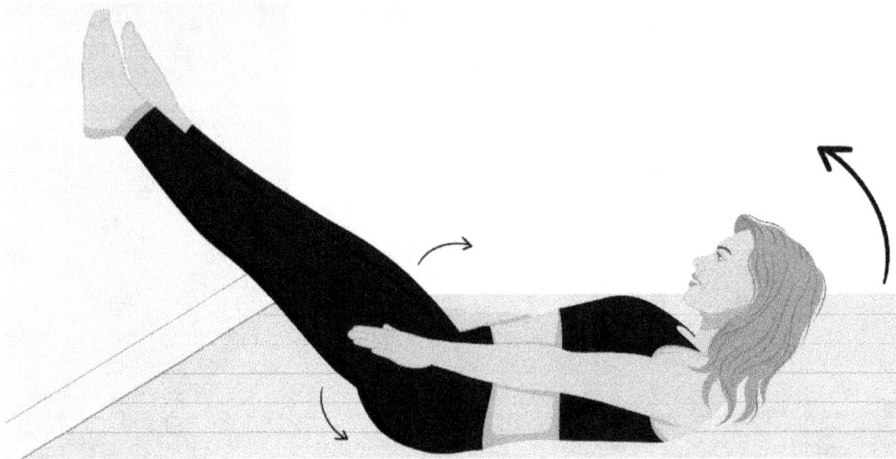

Instructions

- Lie on your back with your legs up the wall, hips close to the baseboard, and your legs straight up the wall.
- Lift your head, neck, and shoulders slightly off the floor, press your back into the ground.
- Extend your arms alongside your body, hovering a few inches off the floor, palms down.
- Engage your core by pulling your navel towards your spine.
- Begin pulsing your arms up and down about 2-3 inches, keeping them straight.
- As you pulse, breathe in for five counts and out for five counts.
- Continue this movement and breathing pattern for 1 minute.

Modifications

- Easier: Keep your head on the floor if lifting it causes neck strain, or bend your knees slightly against the wall.
- Harder: Move your hips a few inches away from the wall, maintaining the leg position without wall support.
- Props: Hold light weights or small water bottles in your hands for added upper-body engagement.

Tips

- Keep your core engaged throughout the exercise to protect your lower back.
- Maintain a consistent, controlled pulse with your arms.
- Focus on deep, rhythmic breathing coordinated with your arm movements.
- Keep your shoulders down and away from your ears.

Wall Pilates Routine: Days 12-14

Warm-up: 2 minutes

1. Forward Lunge: 1 minute
2. Shoulder Press: 1 minute
3. Wall Squats: 1 minute
4. Wall Figure Four: 30 seconds on each side
5. Wall Bridge: 1 minute
6. Single Leg Stretch: 30 seconds on each side
7. Wall Marches: 1 minute
8. 100s: 1 minute

Now that you've gone through Week 2, you're ready to deepen your wall Pilates workout further in Week 3.

CHAPTER 6
WEEK 3—DEEPENING PILATES WORKOUT

*A*s you begin Week 3 of your wall Pilates journey, it's time to take your practice to new depths, building upon the strong foundation you established. This week, your focus will be cultivating deeper muscle engagement, refining your control, and introducing balance challenges and dynamic movements to enhance your mind-body connection and overall fitness.

Emphasis on Deeper Muscle Engagement and Control

This week, the emphasis will be on deeper muscle engagement and control, recruiting those deeper, stabilizing muscles that often get overshadowed by their bigger counterparts: the transverse abdominis (the deepest layer of your abs), the multifidus (the little muscles along your spine), and the pelvic floor (essential for core stability). These muscles play a crucial role in maintaining proper alignment, preventing injury, and creating a solid foundation for all your movements.

By focusing on deeper muscle engagement, you're not only strengthening these muscles but also learning how to control and coordinate them more effectively. In your Week 3 workouts, you will target these deeper muscle groups through exercises requiring greater precision, balance, and body awareness.

Exploring Balance Challenges and Dynamic Movements

Balance challenges are an essential aspect of our Week 3 workouts, as they help to develop your proprioception (the body's ability to sense its position in space), coordination, and functional strength. By intentionally challenging your balance and stability muscles, you better prepare yourself for the demands of daily life, such as navigating uneven surfaces or reaching for objects overhead. Dynamic movements, which emphasize flow, fluidity, and functional range of motion, complement the more static, isolated exercises typically associated with wall Pilates. These dynamic exercises help to improve flexibility and mobility and train your muscles to work together more efficiently and effectively, promoting a more well-rounded and functional approach to fitness.

As you progress through Week 3, it's crucial to remember that growth often occurs outside of your comfort zone, and each challenge you face is an opportunity to celebrate your body's remarkable capabilities. Wall pilates is a practice that continually evolves and grows with you, regardless of your starting point. Every time you show up to your mat, you can deepen your mind-body connection and unlock new levels of strength and potential. Embrace the progression, trust the process, and approach each new challenge with excitement and curiosity, knowing that every shake and victory is proof of your dedication and resilience.

Day 15 to 18: Wall Pilates Exercises

Wall Plank

Wall Planks strengthen the core, improve posture, and engage the shoulders and back muscles. This exercise is excellent for building isometric strength and stability.

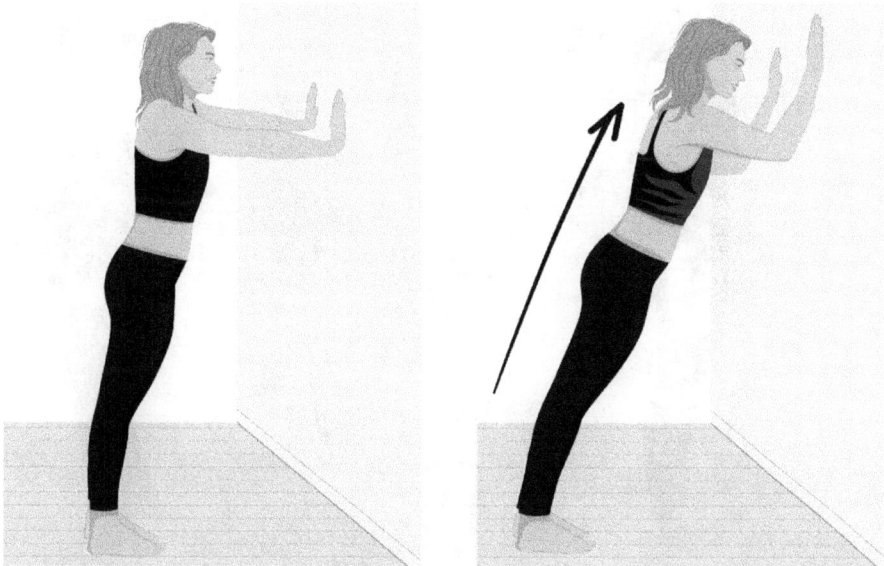

Instructions

- Stand facing a wall, about arm's length away.
- Place your palms flat against the wall at shoulder height.
- Step your feet back, leaning against the wall, and draw a straight line from your head to your heels.
- Keep your core engaged and your body straight, similar to a regular plank position.
- Hold this position for 1 minute.

Modifications

- Easier: Move your feet closer to the wall to reduce the angle and difficulty.
- Harder: Step your feet further away from the wall to increase the angle and challenge.
- Props: Place a yoga block between your hands to engage your chest muscles more.

Tips

- Keep your neck aligned with your spine, avoiding dropping or lifting your head.
- Engage your glutes and quad muscles to maintain a straight body line.
- Breathe steadily throughout the hold.
- If you feel wrist discomfort, try making fists against the wall instead of using flat palms.

Standing Wall Roll-Down

Standing Wall Roll-Downs improve spinal flexibility, stretch the back muscles, and promote better posture. This exercise helps decompress the spine and release tension.

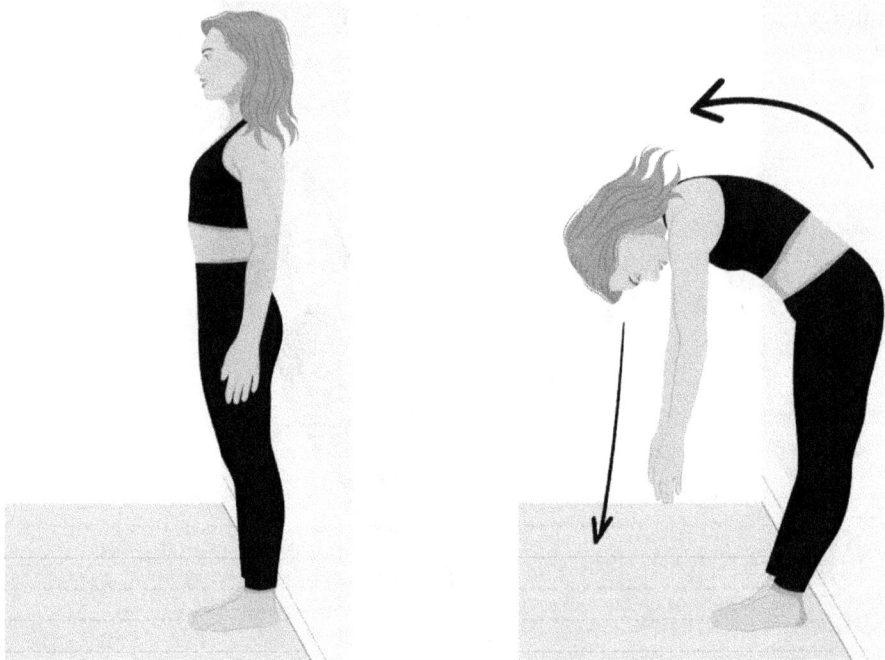

Instructions

- Stand with your back against a wall, feet hip-width apart and about 6 inches from the wall.
- Start by tucking your chin to your chest.
- Slowly roll down, peeling your spine away from the wall vertebra by vertebra.
- Continue rolling down as far as comfortable, letting your arms hang towards the floor.
- Hold the bottom position for a moment, then slowly roll back up to the starting position.
- Repeat this movement for 1 minute.

Modifications

- Easier: Don't roll down as far, focusing on the upper and mid-back areas.
- Harder: Hold the bottom position for longer before rolling back up.
- Props: Place a small cushion behind your lower back for support if needed.

Tips

- Move slowly and deliberately, focusing on each vertebra as you roll down and up.
- Breathe steadily, exhaling as you roll down and inhaling as you roll up.
- If you feel any pain or discomfort, especially in your lower back, reduce your range of motion.

Wall Pike Pushup

This exercise targets your shoulders, upper chest, and core while improving balance and body awareness.

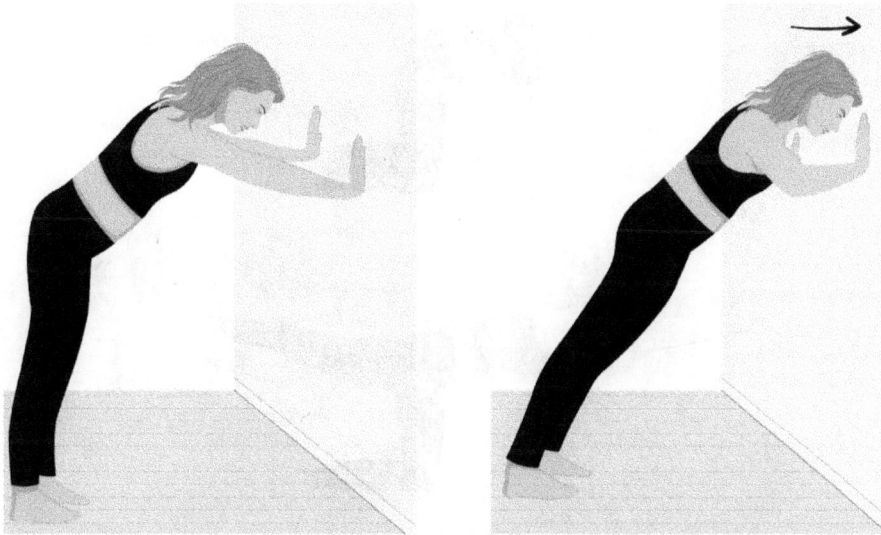

Instructions:

- Stand facing a wall, about arm's length away.
- Place your hands on the wall at shoulder height and shoulder width apart.
- Walk your feet back while sliding your hands down the wall until your body forms an inverted "V" shape.
- Your head should be between your arms, your heels lifted, and your body straight from your hands to your hips.
- Slowly bend your elbows, lowering your upper body to move towards the wall while maintaining the "V" shape in your body.
- Push back up to the starting position, fully extending your arms. Repeat for 1 minute.

Modifications:

- Easier: Keep your feet closer to the wall for a less intense angle.
- Harder: Walk your feet further from the wall to increase the angle and difficulty.
- Props: Use yoga blocks under your hands for an increased range of motion.

Tips:

- Keep your body in a straight line from hands to hips.

Wall Bird Dog

This exercise enhances core stability, improves balance, and strengthens the back and hips muscles.

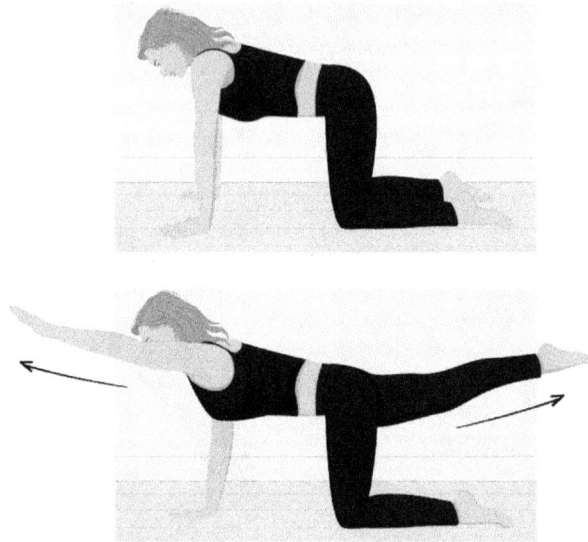

Instructions:

- Enter into a tabletop position with your right shoulder touching the wall and your right hip about 6 inches from the wall.
- Stack your hands under your shoulders and your knees under your hips.
- Engage your core and keep your spine neutral.
- Slowly lift your left arm off the floor and extend it parallel to the ground.
- At the same time, lift your right foot off the floor and extend your leg back.
- Hold this position for 2-3 seconds, focusing on balance and stability.
- Return to the starting position and repeat your movement for 30 seconds.
- Once you've completed the exercise, turn around so that your left shoulder touches the wall and perform the exercise on the other side for 30 seconds.

Modifications:

- Easier: Keep your shoulder and hips against the wall for support.
- Harder: Increase the hold time to 5-10 seconds for each repetition.
- Props: Place a small pillow or folded towel under your knees for additional cushioning.

Tips:

- Breathe steadily: inhale as you extend, exhale as you return to the starting position.
- Maintain a straight line from your head to your heels throughout the movement.
- If you feel any lower back strain, reduce the range of motion or return to the starting position.
- Gaze at a fixed point on the wall to help maintain balance.

Alternate Leg Flexion

Alternate Leg Flexion improves hip flexibility, strengthens the core, and enhances lower-body coordination.

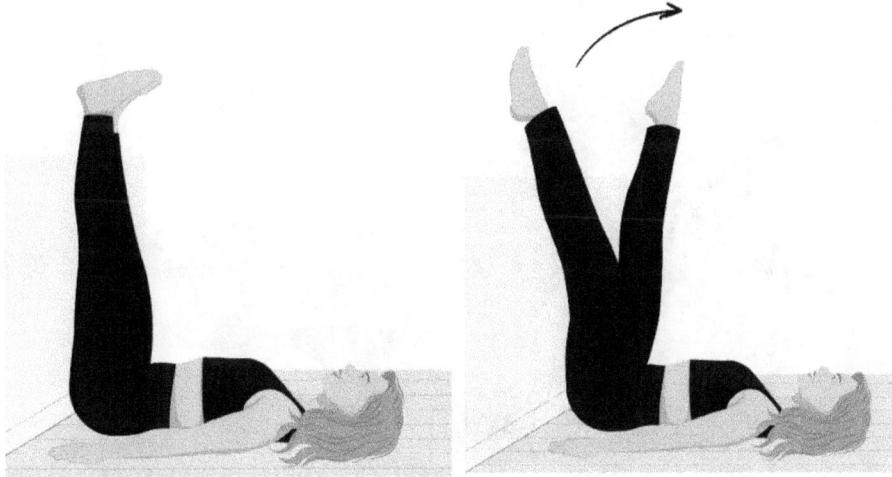

Instructions

- Lie on your back on the floor with your buttocks close to a wall, about 6 inches away.
- Extend both legs up the wall, bending your knees.
- Your body should form an inverted L shape, with your back on the floor and legs up the wall.
- Keep your upper back, shoulders, and head in contact with the floor throughout the exercise.
- Place your arms at your sides, palms down, for stability.
- Lift your right foot off the wall, moving your thigh towards your chest.
- Hold for 2-3 seconds, then slowly move your right foot back to the wall.
- Lift your left foot in the same manner.
- Continue alternating legs for 1 minute.

Modifications

- Easier: Make smaller movements or slightly bend your knee.
- Harder: Hold each leg lift for 5 seconds before switching.
- Props: Use a small pillow under your lower back if you feel pain or discomfort.

Tips

- Keep your core engaged throughout the exercise to support your lower back.
- Maintain contact between your upper back and the floor during the entire movement.

Wall-Assisted Bicycle

This exercise targets your core muscles, particularly the obliques, while engaging the hip flexors and improving coordination.

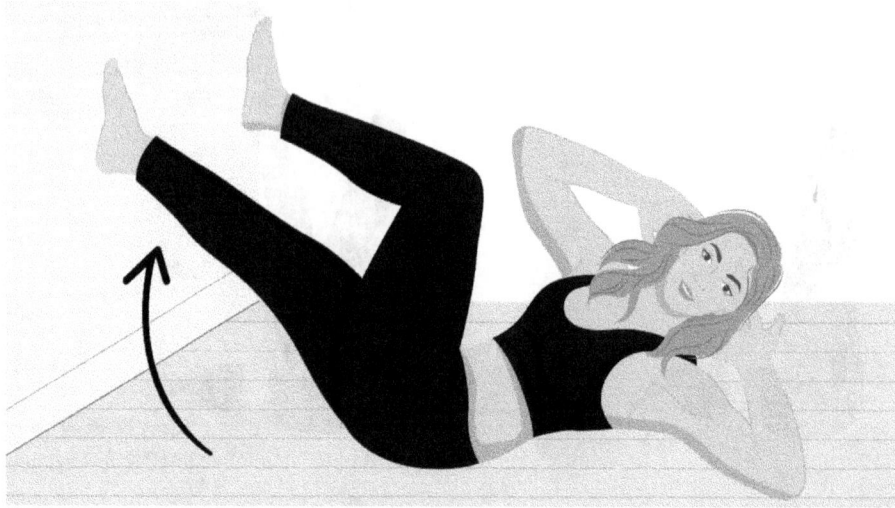

Instructions:

- Lie on your back with your buttocks close to the wall legs extended up the wall.
- Place your hands behind your head, elbows pointing outward.
- Lift your shoulders slightly off the ground, engaging your upper abdominals.
- Bend your right knee and slide your right foot down the wall while simultaneously extending your left leg up the wall.
- As you do this, rotate your upper body to bring your left elbow towards your right knee.
- Return to the center and repeat on the other side, bending your left knee and rotating to bring your right elbow towards it.
- Continue alternating sides in a fluid, cycling motion for 1 minute.

Modifications:

- Easier: Keep your head and shoulders on the ground and focus on the leg movements.
- Harder: Increase speed while maintaining control or add a pause at each rotation.
- Props: Use a yoga mat for cushioning under your back if needed.

Tips:

- Keep your lower back pressed against the floor throughout the exercise.
- Breathe steadily: exhale as you rotate, inhale as you return to the center.
- Focus on the rotation coming from your core, not just moving your elbows.
- Maintain a consistent, controlled pace rather than rushing through the movements.
- If you feel neck strain, support your head lightly with your hands; don't pull on it.

Wall Scissors

This exercise targets your lower abdominal muscles and hip flexors and improves core stability.

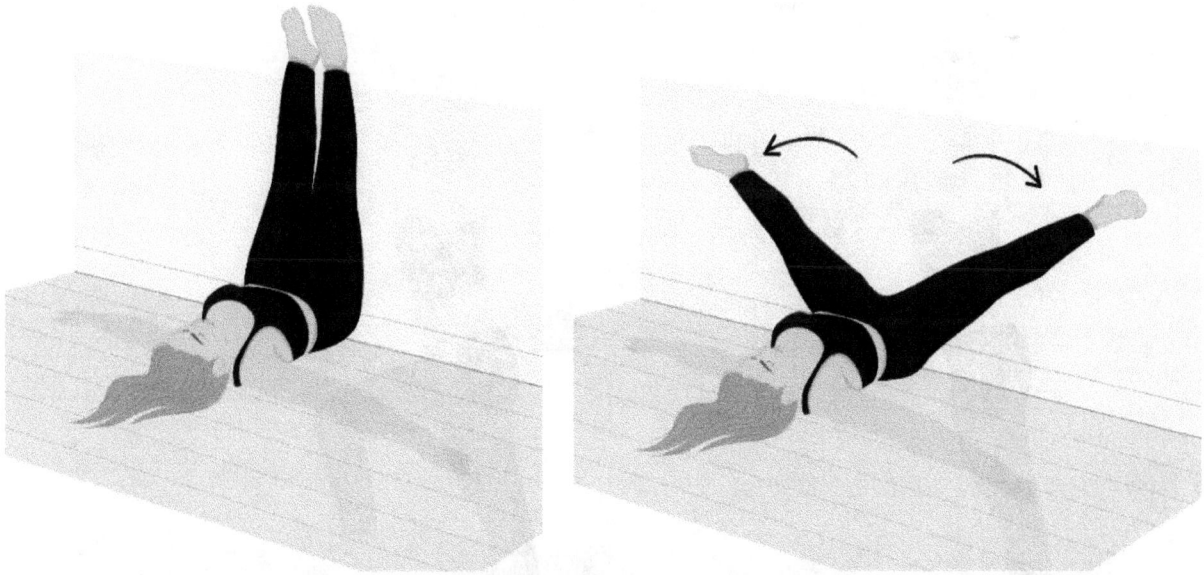

Instructions:

- Lie on your back with your buttocks close to a wall, legs extended up the wall.
- Place your arms at your sides, palms down, for stability.
- Engage your core by pressing your lower back into the floor.
- Slowly lower your right and left legs down the wall, keeping them straight, in a "V" position.
- Keep your back flat, and slowly bring your legs back together.
- Continue this alternating scissors-like motion, keeping both legs straight for 1 minute.

Modifications:

- Easier: Reduce the range of motion, not lowering your legs as far down the wall.
- Harder: Increase speed while maintaining control, or hold your head and shoulders slightly off the ground.
- Props: Use a small pillow under your head for neck support if needed.

Tips:

- Keep your movements slow and controlled to maximize muscle engagement.
- Maintain constant contact between your lower back and the floor throughout the exercise.
- If you feel any strain in your lower back, reduce the range of motion or bend your knees slightly.
- Focus on using your core muscles to control the leg movements rather than relying on momentum.

Wall Mountain Climbers

Wall Mountain Climbers provide a low-impact cardiovascular workout while engaging the core, hip flexors, and legs.

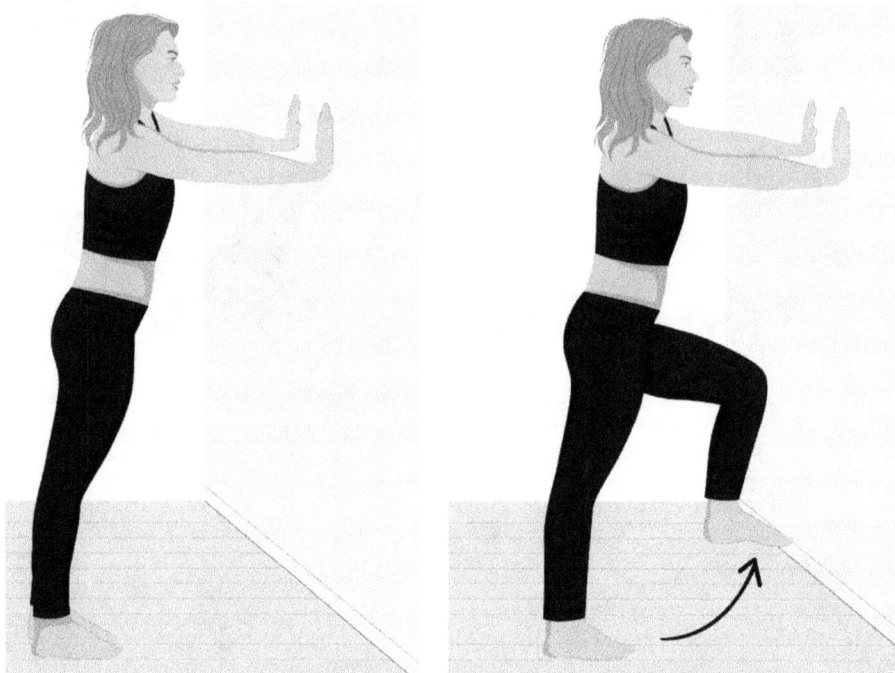

Instructions

- Start in a wall plank position, hands against the wall at shoulder height, body in a straight line.
- Bring your right knee to your chest, then return it to the starting position.
- Immediately bring your left knee up towards your chest, then return it.
- Continue alternating legs in a running motion.
- Perform this exercise for 1 minute.

Modifications

- Easier: Perform the movement more slowly or bring your knees up to a lower height.
- Harder: Increase the speed of the movement, raise your legs higher, or step your feet further away from the wall.
- Props: Place sliders or small towels under your feet to reduce friction with the floor.

Tips

- Keep your core engaged throughout the exercise to maintain a straight body line.
- Breathe steadily, finding a rhythm with your movements.

Wall Pilates Routine: Day 15-18

Warm-Up: 2 minutes

1. Wall Plank: 1 minute
2. Standing Wall Roll-Down: 1 minute
3. Wall Pike Pushup: 1 minute
4. Wall Bird Dog: 30 seconds on each side
5. Alternate Leg Flexion: 30 seconds on each side
6. Wall-Assisted Bicycle: 1 minute
7. Wall Scissors: 30 seconds on each side
8. Wall Mountain Climbers: 1 minute

Incorporating More Advanced Breathwork

Before continuing with week 3, let's explore one more powerful breathing exercise that can enhance your practice and deepen your mind-body connection. Incorporating this technique into your daily routine can help improve rib cage mobility, target hard-to-reach back muscles, and promote relaxation and stress relief.

While you should now be familiar with lateral breathing, this breathwork practice can be expanded upon to use posterior lateral breathing. This variation of traditional lateral breathing emphasizes expanding the back and sides of your ribcage.

As you inhale, focus on expanding the back and sides of your rib cage rather than the front. A great way to test this is to lie on the floor or your mat and attempt posterior lateral breath. If your back lifts slightly off the mat, you are breathing laterally and posteriorly.

This exercise is particularly beneficial for targeting those hard-to-reach back muscles that can become tight and tense after long hours hunched over a desk or engaged in other sedentary activities. As you incorporate these breathing exercises into your wall Pilates practice, take the time to tune into your body's sensations and respond to its unique needs.

Day 19 to 21: Wall Pilates Exercises

Forward Lunge

Forward Wall Lunges strengthen the quadriceps, hamstrings, and glutes while improving balance and hip mobility.

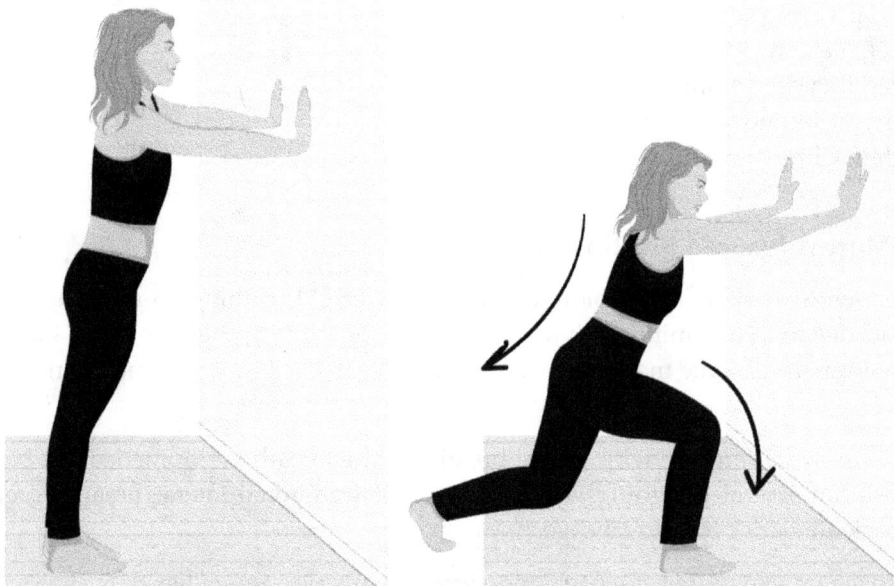

Instructions

- Stand facing the wall, about arm's length away.
- Place your palms flat against the wall at chest height for support.
- Take a large step forward with your right foot, keeping your left foot in place.
- Bend both knees to lower your body, keeping your front knee aligned over your ankle.
- Lower yourself until your back knee is a few inches from the ground or as far as comfortable.
- Push through your front heel to return to the starting position.
- Repeat with the left leg stepping forward.
- Continue alternating legs for 1 minute.

Modifications

- Easier: Start closer to the wall, take a smaller step forward, and don't lower as deeply.
- Harder: Hold the lunge position for 2-3 seconds before pushing back up, or add a knee lift with the front leg before stepping forward.
- Props: Hold light dumbbells at your sides for added resistance.

Tips

- Keep your chest up and shoulders back, avoiding leaning into the wall.

Arm Slides

Arm Slides improve shoulder mobility, engage the core, and strengthen the upper body while promoting good posture.

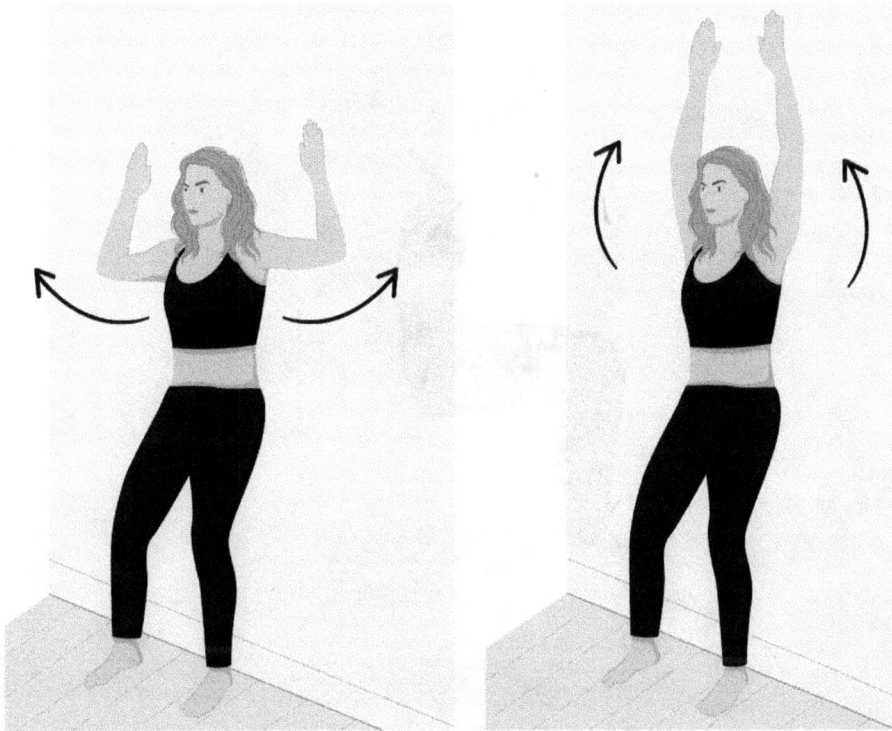

Instructions

- Stand with your back against a wall, feet about 6 inches from the base.
- Press your entire back, arms, and hands against the wall, with your arms at your sides.
- Slowly slide your arms up the wall until they're straight overhead.
- Hold briefly, then slide them back down to the starting position.
- Repeat this movement for 1 minute.

Modifications

- Easier: Only slide your arms up halfway if the full overhead extension is challenging.
- Harder: Hold light weights while performing the movement or pause for longer at the top.
- Props: Use small towels under your hands to allow them to slide more easily against the wall.

Tips

- Keep your lower back pressed against the wall throughout the movement.
- Focus on keeping your shoulders down and away from your ears.
- If you feel any shoulder discomfort, reduce your range of motion.

Wall Sit with Squat Pulse

This exercise combines the isometric hold of a wall sit with dynamic squatting pulses, targeting your quadriceps, glutes, and calves.

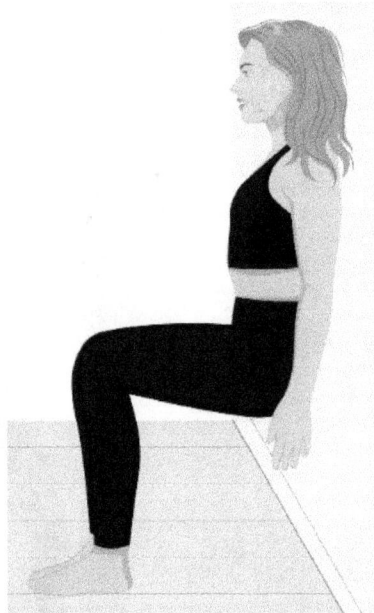

Instructions:

- Stand with your back against a wall, feet shoulder-width apart and about 2 feet away from the wall.
- Slowly slide your back down the wall until your thighs parallel the ground, forming a 90-degree angle at your knees.
- Your knees should be directly above your ankles, not extending past your toes.
- Hold this position, keeping your back flat against the wall.
- From this wall sit position, begin small pulsing movements up and down.
- Continue these pulsing movements for 1 minute.

Modifications:

- Easier: Hold the wall sit for a shorter duration or reduce the number of pulses.
- Harder: Hold light weights in each hand.
- Props: Place a small exercise ball between your back and the wall for comfort and feedback.

Tips:

- Keep your core engaged throughout the exercise to support your lower back.
- Breathe steadily: avoid holding your breath during the hold or pulses.
- Ensure your feet are far enough from the wall so your knees don't extend past your toes.

Leaning Hip Circles

This exercise improves core strength, spinal mobility, and hip flexibility.

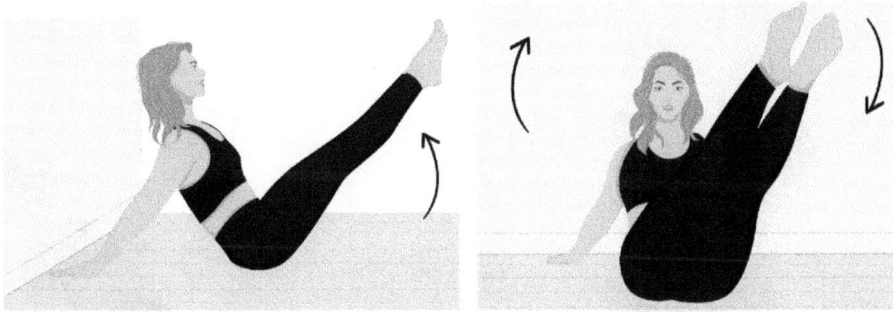

<u>Instructions:</u>

- Sit with your back to the wall about an arm's length away.
- Bend your knees and place your hands behind you so that your fingertips touch the wall.
- Use the wall as support by making contact with your shoulders if you would like.
- Engage your core and lift both legs off the floor, straightening them if possible.
- Slowly rotate your legs in a clockwise motion for 30 seconds.
- Place your feet back on the mat to recenter yourself.
- When you are ready, lift both legs off the floor once more and rotate them counterclockwise for 30 seconds.

<u>Modifications:</u>

- Easier: Reduce the range of motion in the circles.
- Harder: Lift the foot farthest from the wall off the ground as you twist, balancing on one leg.
- Props: If you have difficulty reaching the wall comfortably, put a yoga block between your hand and the wall.

<u>Tips:</u>

- Keep your supporting arm slightly bent to avoid locking the elbow.
- Breathe steadily: inhale as you prepare, exhale as you twist, and inhale to return.
- Maintain a stable lower body; the rotation should come from your spine and core.
- Keep your hips facing forward throughout the movement.

Single-Leg Glute Bridge

This exercise targets the glutes, hamstrings, and core muscles while improving hip stability and lower body strength.

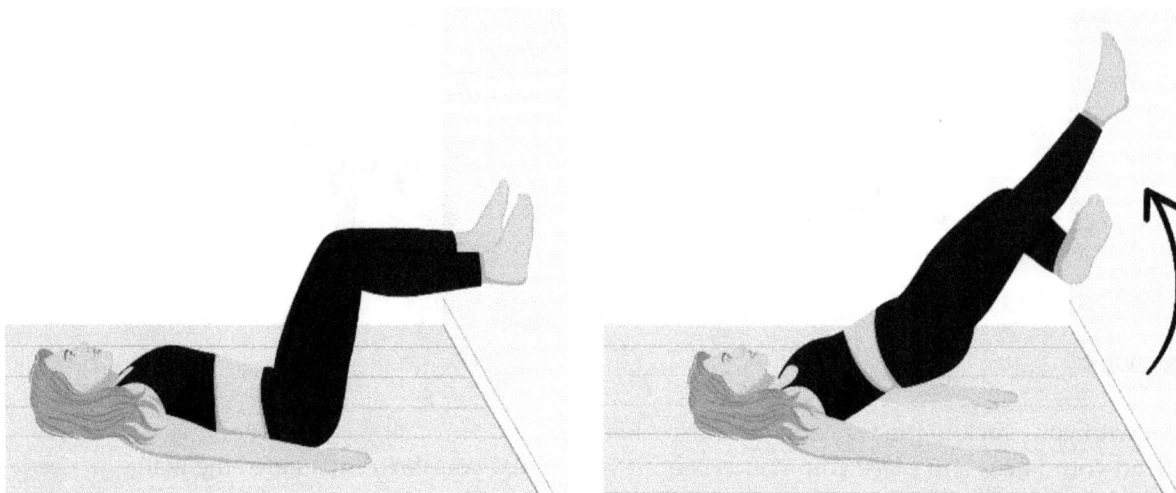

Instructions:

- Lie on your back with your knees bent and feet flat on the wall, hip-width apart.
- Place your arms at your sides, palms down, for stability, or on your hips, whichever is more comfortable for you.
- Engage your core and squeeze your glutes to lift your hips.
- Raise your hips until your body forms a straight line from your left knee to your shoulders.
- Tuck your left foot under your right leg without allowing it to touch the mat.
- Hold this position for 30 seconds.
- Slowly lower your hips back to the starting position.
- Perform the exercise on the other side for 30 seconds.

Modifications:

- Easier: Keep both feet on the wall and perform a standard glute bridge.
- Harder: Place your supporting foot on an elevated surface like a low step or yoga block.
- Props: Use a resistance band around your thighs just above the knees for added challenge.

Tips:

- Keep your raised leg straight and aligned with your body throughout the movement.
- Maintain a neutral spine; avoid arching your lower back as you lift.
- Focus on pushing through the heel of the supporting foot to engage your glutes fully.
- Keep your hips level as you lift; don't let the hip of your raised leg drop.

Supine Side Bend

This gentle, restorative pose helps improve spinal mobility, stretches the back muscles, and releases tension in the lower back.

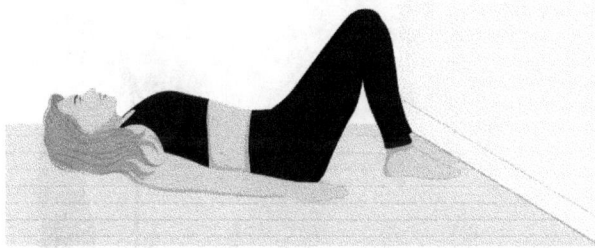

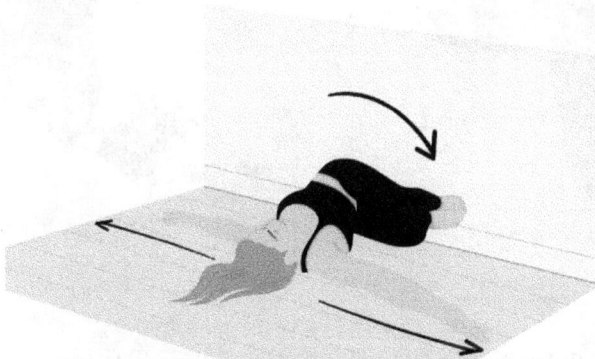

Instructions:

- Lie on your back with your knees bent and feet flat on the floor, touching the wall.
- Place your arms out straight at your sides with palms facing down.
- Slowly lower your knees to the right, keeping both shoulders flat on the floor.
- Allow your knees to rest on the floor (or as close as comfortable).
- Hold this position for 30 seconds, breathing deeply.
- Slowly return your legs to the starting position.
- Repeat on the other side for 30 seconds.

Modifications:

- Easier: Place a pillow or folded blanket under your buttocks for support.
- Harder: Extend your top leg straight while keeping the bottom leg bent.
- Props: Use a bolster or firm pillow under your knees for added comfort.

Tips:

- If your knees don't reach the floor, that's okay. Only go as far as is comfortable.
- Keep both shoulders pressed into the floor to maintain the spinal twist.

Single-Leg Stretch

Single-Leg Stretches improve hamstring flexibility, strengthen the core, and enhance balance. This exercise targets multiple muscle groups simultaneously.

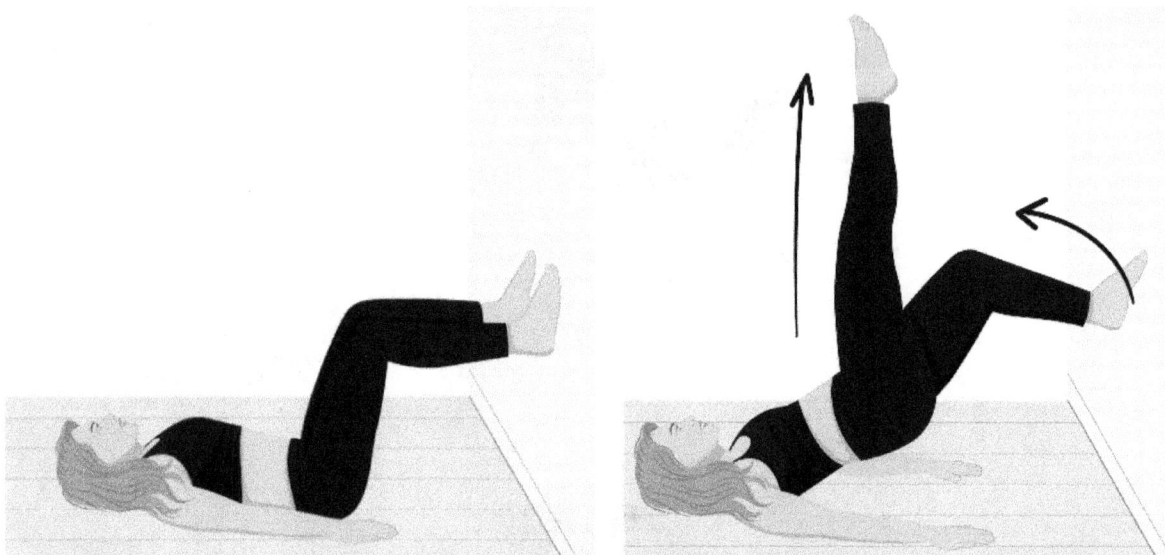

Instructions

- Lie on your back with both legs extended and resting on the wall with your knees bent.
- Lift your right leg and straighten it.
- Slowly lift your right leg toward the ceiling until you feel the stretch in your hamstring.
- If you find it challenging to keep your leg lifted unassisted, feel free to use your right hand to grip the back of your thigh for support gently.
- Hold for 30 seconds, then slowly lower the leg.
- Switch sides and repeat with the left leg for 30 seconds.

Modifications

- Easier: Bend your knee slightly if you can't keep your leg straight.
- Harder: Lift your head and shoulders off the ground to engage your core more.
- Props: Use a yoga strap around your foot to help pull your leg closer if you can't reach your ankle.

Tips

- Keep your lower back pressed into the floor throughout the movement.
- If you feel any strain in your lower back, bend your knee more or reduce the stretch.
- Breathe deeply and evenly, focusing on relaxing into the stretch.

100s

Wall 100s intensely engage the core muscles, particularly the lower abdominals, while using the wall for leg support.

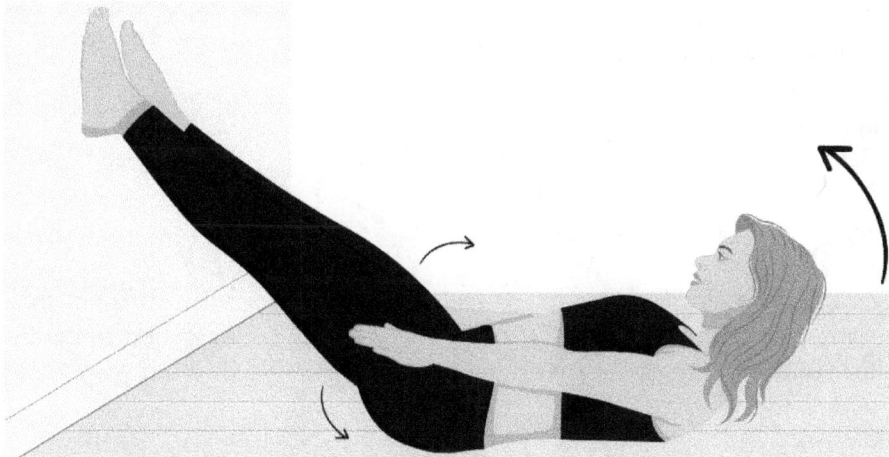

Instructions

- Lie on your back with your legs up the wall, hips close to the baseboard, and your legs straight up the wall.
- Lift your head, neck, and shoulders slightly off the floor, pressing your lower back into the ground.
- Extend your arms straight alongside your body, hovering a few inches off the floor, palms down.
- Engage your core by pulling your navel towards your spine.
- Begin pulsing your arms up and down about 2-3 inches, keeping them straight.
- As you pulse, breathe in for five counts and out for five counts.
- Continue this movement and breathing pattern for 1 minute.

Modifications

- Easier: Keep your head on the floor if lifting it causes neck strain, or bend your knees slightly against the wall.
- Harder: Move your hips a few inches away from the wall, maintaining the leg position without wall support.
- Props: Hold light weights in your hands for added upper-body engagement.

Tips

- Keep your core engaged throughout the exercise to protect your lower back.
- Maintain a consistent, controlled pulse with your arms.
- Keep your shoulders down and away from your ears.

Wall Pilates Routine Day 19-21

Warm-Up: 2 minutes

1. Forward Lunge: 1 minute
2. Arm Slides: 1 minute
3. Wall Sit with Squat Pulse: 1 minute
4. Leaning Hip Circles: 30 seconds on each side
5. Single Leg Glute Bridge: 30 seconds on each side
6. Supine Side Bend: 1 minute
7. Single Leg Stretch: 30 seconds on each side
8. 100s: 1 minute

After completing week 3's exercises, you might feel your muscles a little stiff, but this is entirely normal and just a sign that your muscles are adapting and growing stronger. Remember that rest days are as necessary for your recovery as your workouts, nutrition, and hydration. Always listen to your body, and factor in time to rest.

That said, it is time to enter the fourth and final week of your wall Pilates journey.

CHAPTER 7
WEEK 4—MASTERING WALL PILATES

*A*s you step into Week 4 of your wall Pilates journey, it's time to embrace the complex, multi-layered movements that truly showcase the beauty, artistry, and total-body transformation that this practice offers.

Mastering wall Pilates techniques is not merely about learning new exercises for the sake of novelty. Integrating all the skills, techniques, and principles you've acquired into a fluid, harmonious, and highly effective wall Pilates practice that will leave you feeling like the strongest, most graceful version of yourself. This mastery is rooted in refinement, precision, and a heightened sense of body awareness, allowing you to move with intention and control.

Throughout the Week 4 workouts, you'll be challenged to engage multiple muscle groups simultaneously, creating a symphony of movement that showcases Pilates's true power and potential. However, it's crucial to remember that mastery is not about perfection—the journey, the process, and the unwavering commitment to growth and self-improvement.

Day 22 to 25: Wall Pilates Workouts

Wall Plank

Wall Planks strengthen the core, improve posture, and engage the shoulders and back muscles. This exercise is excellent for building isometric strength and stability.

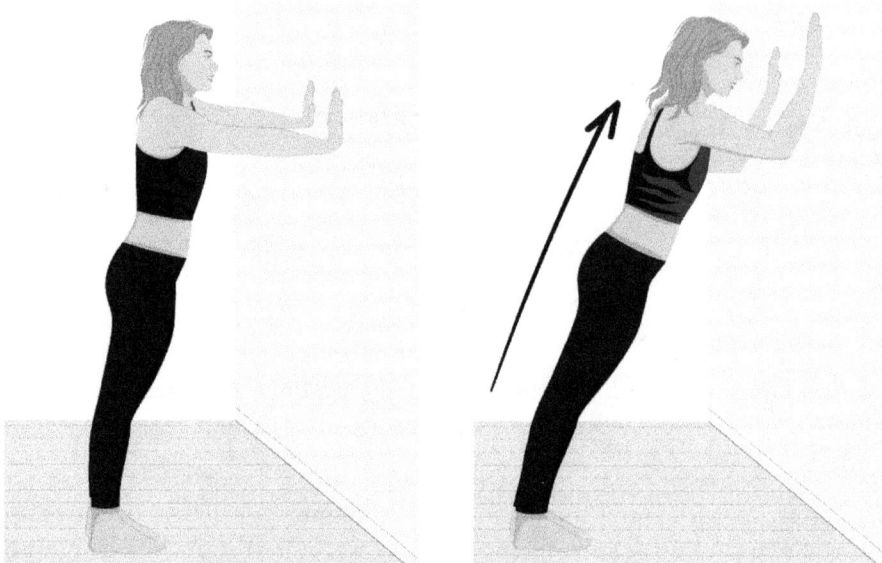

Instructions

- Stand facing a wall, about arm's length away.
- Place your palms flat against the wall at shoulder height.
- Step your feet back, leaning against the wall, and draw a straight line from your head to your heels.
- Keep your core engaged and your body straight, similar to a regular plank position.
- Hold this position for 1 minute.

Modifications

- Easier: Move your feet closer to the wall to reduce the angle and difficulty.
- Harder: Step your feet further away from the wall to increase the angle and challenge.
- Props: Place a yoga block between your hands to engage your chest muscles more.

Tips

- Keep your neck aligned with your spine, avoiding dropping or lifting your head.
- Engage your glutes and quad muscles to maintain a straight body line.
- Breathe steadily throughout the hold.
- If you feel wrist discomfort, try making fists against the wall instead of using flat palms.

Plank to Wall Tap

This exercise enhances core stability, upper body strength, and coordination.

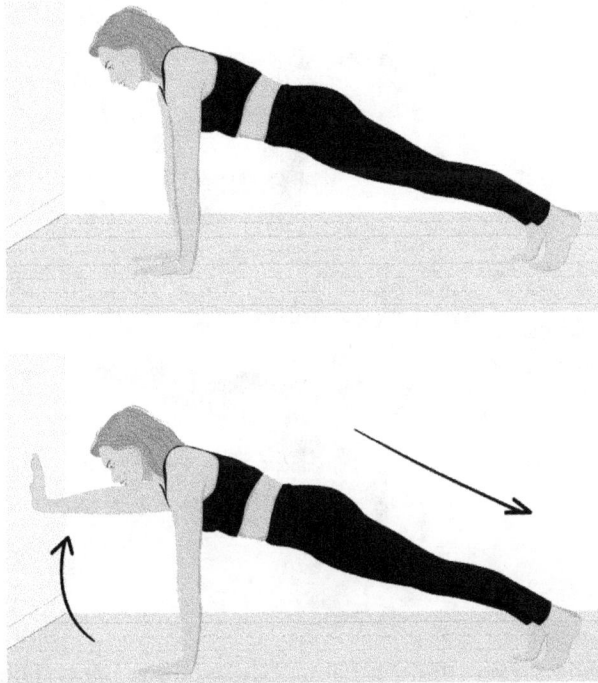

Instructions:

- Start in a plank position with your head facing the wall. Hands stacked under your shoulders.
- Your feet should be shoulder-width apart on the floor, and your body should form a straight line from head to heels.
- Engage your core, glutes, and thighs, lift your left hand onto the wall at about chest height and your right hand on the floor.
- Lower your left hand back to the mat and re-enter into a plank position.
- Engage your core, glutes, and thighs once more, and lift your right hand onto the wall.
- Continue to alternate arm touches for 1 minute.

Modifications:

- Easier: Place your hand higher on the wall to decrease the angle of your body.
- Harder: Place your hand lower on the wall to increase the angle and difficulty.
- Props: Use a yoga mat under your floor for comfort.

Tips:

- Keep your body in a straight line throughout the exercise; don't let your hips rotate or sag.

Wall Bird Dog

This exercise enhances core stability, improves balance, and strengthens the back and hips muscles.

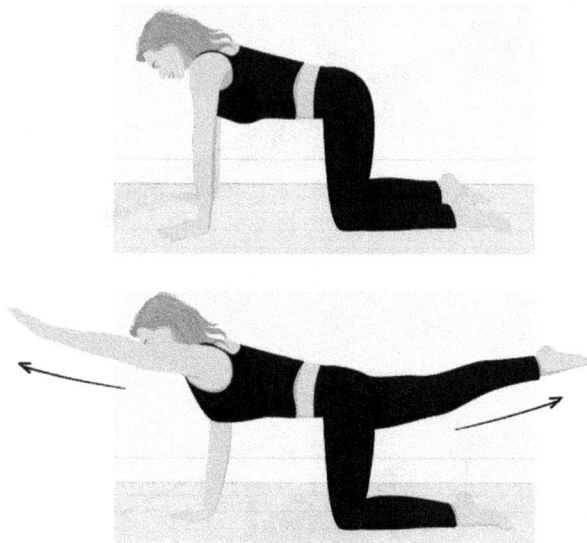

Instructions:

- Enter into a tabletop position with your right shoulder touching the wall and your right hip about 6 inches from the wall.
- Stack your hands under your shoulders and your knees under your hips.
- Engage your core and keep your spine neutral.
- Slowly lift your left arm off the floor and extend it parallel to the ground.
- At the same time, lift your right foot off the floor and extend your leg back.
- Hold this position for 2-3 seconds, focusing on balance and stability.
- Return to the starting position and repeat your movement for 30 seconds.
- Once you've completed the exercise, turn around so that your left shoulder touches the wall and perform the exercise on the other side for 30 seconds.

Modifications:

- Easier: Keep your shoulder and hips against the wall for support.
- Harder: Increase the hold time to 5-10 seconds for each repetition.
- Props: Place a small pillow or folded towel under your knees for additional cushioning.

Tips:

- Keep your movements slow and controlled throughout the exercise.
- Breathe steadily: inhale as you extend, exhale as you return to the starting position.
- Maintain a straight line from your head to your heels throughout the movement.
- Gaze at a fixed point on the wall to help maintain balance.

Wall-Assisted Bicycle

This exercise targets your core muscles, particularly the obliques, while engaging the hip flexors and improving coordination.

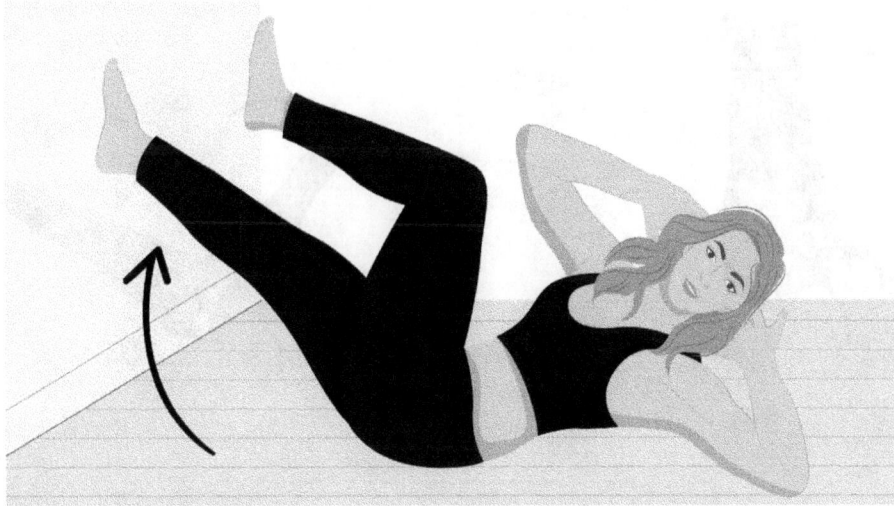

Instructions:

- Lie on your back with your buttocks close to the wall legs extended up the wall.
- Place your hands behind your head, elbows pointing outward.
- Lift your shoulders slightly off the ground, engaging your upper abdominals.
- Bend your right knee and slide your right foot down the wall while simultaneously extending your left leg up the wall.
- As you do this, rotate your upper body to bring your left elbow towards your right knee.
- Return to the center and repeat on the other side, bending your left knee and rotating to bring your right elbow towards it.
- Continue alternating sides in a fluid, cycling motion for 1 minute.

Modifications:

- Easier: Keep your head and shoulders on the ground and focus on the leg movements.
- Harder: Increase speed while maintaining control or add a pause at each rotation.
- Props: Use a yoga mat for cushioning under your back if needed.

Tips:

- Keep your lower back pressed against the floor throughout the exercise.
- Breathe steadily: exhale as you rotate, inhale as you return to the center.
- Focus on the rotation coming from your core, not just moving your elbows.
- Maintain a consistent, controlled pace rather than rushing through the movements.
- If you feel neck strain, support your head lightly with your hands; don't pull on it.

Wall Scissors

This exercise targets your lower abdominal muscles and hip flexors and improves core stability.

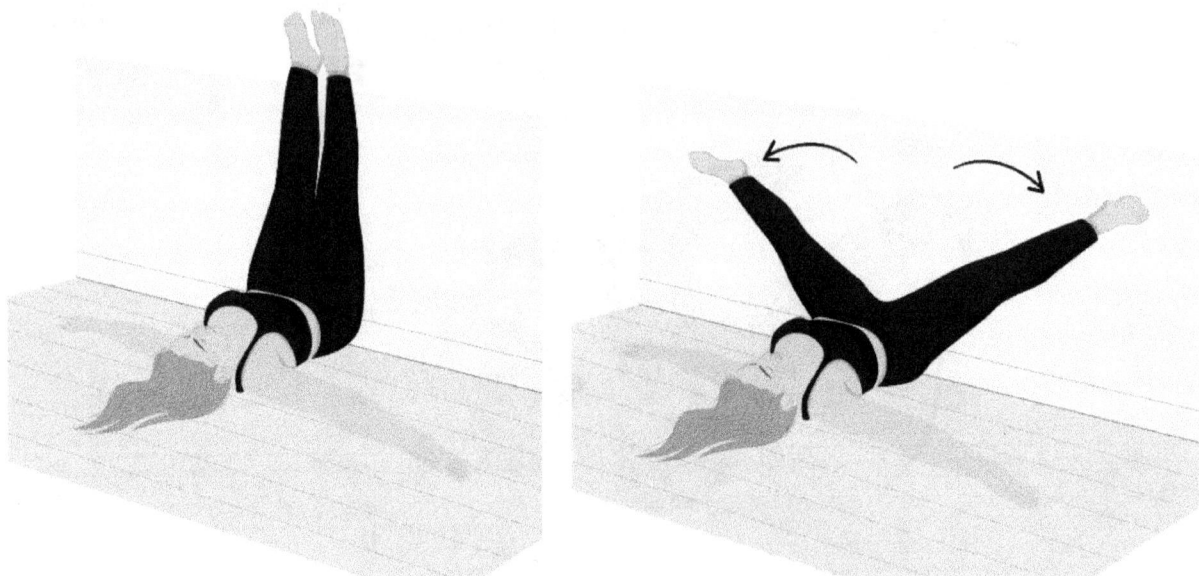

Instructions:

- Lie on your back with your buttocks close to a wall, legs extended up the wall.
- Place your arms at your sides, palms down, for stability.
- Engage your core by pressing your lower back into the floor.
- Slowly lower your right and left legs down the wall, keeping them straight, in a "V" position.
- Keep your back flat, and slowly bring your legs back together.
- Continue this alternating scissors-like motion, keeping both legs straight for 1 minute.

Modifications:

- Easier: Reduce the range of motion, not lowering your legs as far down the wall.
- Harder: Increase speed while maintaining control, or hold your head and shoulders slightly off the ground.
- Props: Use a small pillow under your head for neck support.

Tips:

- Keep your movements slow and controlled to maximize muscle engagement.
- Breathe steadily: exhale as you lower your leg, inhale as you raise it.
- Maintain constant contact between your lower back and the floor throughout the exercise.
- Focus on using your core muscles to control the leg movements rather than relying on momentum.

Boomerang

This wall-supported variation of the Boomerang exercise provides stability while still targeting the core, abdominals, and lower back muscles.

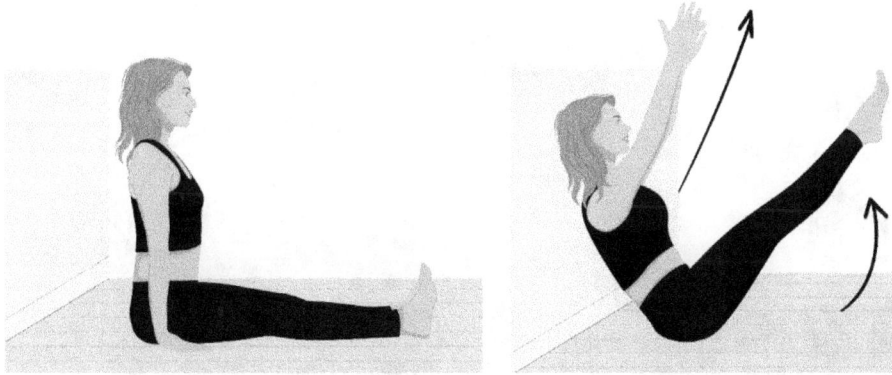

Instructions:

- Start seated on the floor, back about a half arm's length away from the wall, legs extended straight in front of you.
- Lift your arms overhead, reaching towards the ceiling.
- Lean back simultaneously as you lift your legs at about a 45-degree angle, keeping your arms raised.
- Use the wall for support.
- At the top of the movement, your body should form a V-shape, with arms reaching forward parallel to your legs and your upper back still touching the wall.
- Hold this V-position for a moment, then slowly lower back to the starting seated position with your legs back on the ground and your arms close to your legs.
- Repeat this sequence for 1 minute.

Modifications:

- Easier: Keep your knees slightly bent throughout the movement.
- Harder: Hold the V-position at the top for a longer duration.
- Props: Use a yoga mat for comfort on hard floors.

Tips:

- Keep your movements slow and controlled throughout the exercise.
- Breathe steadily: inhale as you slide down, exhale as you slide up.
- Engage your core throughout the entire movement, especially during the V-hold.
- Use the wall as a guide to maintain proper form and alignment.
- Keep your legs together throughout the movement.
- If you feel any neck strain, focus on pressing the back of your head against the wall.

Neck Pull with Wall Touch

This seated exercise targets the deep neck flexors and upper trapezius muscles, improving neck posture and strength.

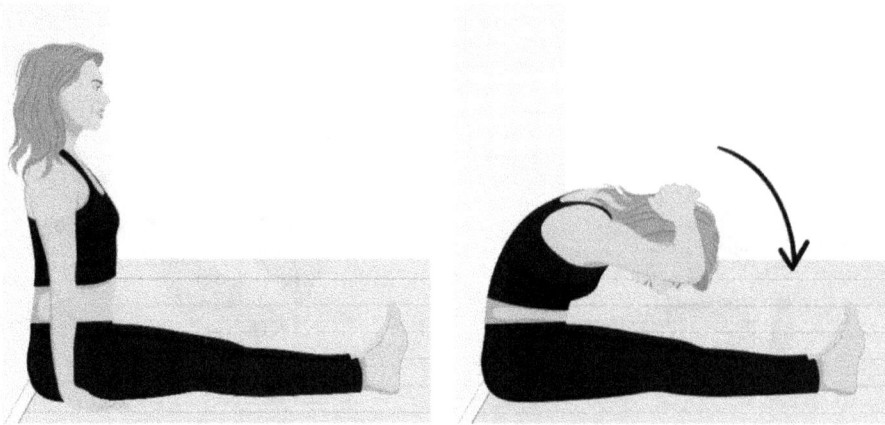

Instructions:

- Sit on the floor with your back against a wall, legs extended straight in front of you.
- Ensure your upper back, shoulders, and head are in contact with the wall.
- Tuck your chin slightly and place your hands behind your head.
- Slowly fold forward at the hips, trying to keep your knees straight.
- Hold this position momentarily before gently putting pressure on your hands by pushing your head up.
- Release the pressure for a moment and then repeat for 1 minute.

Modifications:

- Easier: Bend your knees and place your feet flat on the floor if extending your legs is uncomfortable.
- Harder: Try to place your chest on your thighs.
- Props: Use a yoga mat or folded towel for comfort on hard floors.

Tips:

- Keep the movement slow and controlled throughout the exercise.
- Breathe steadily: inhale as you slide up, exhale as you return to the starting position.
- Maintain contact with the wall throughout the entire movement.
- Focus on creating length in the back of your neck rather than pushing your head back forcefully.
- Stop the exercise if you feel any pain or discomfort, especially a sharp or pinching sensation.

Wall Mountain Climbers

Wall Mountain Climbers provide a low-impact cardiovascular workout while engaging the core, hip flexors, and legs.

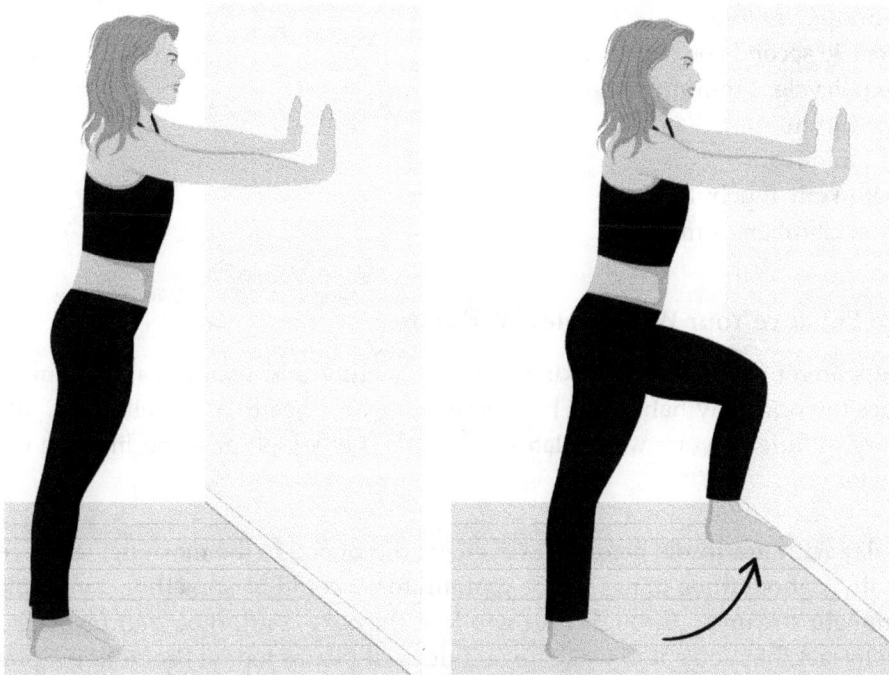

<u>Instructions</u>

- Start in a wall plank position, hands against the wall at shoulder height, body in a straight line.
- Bring your right knee to your chest, then return it to the starting position.
- Immediately bring your left knee up towards your chest, then return it.
- Continue alternating legs in a running motion.
- Perform this exercise for 1 minute.

<u>Modifications</u>

- Easier: Perform the movement more slowly or bring your knees up to a lower height.
- Harder: Increase the speed of the movement, raise your legs higher, or step your feet further away from the wall.
- Props: Place sliders or small towels under your feet to reduce friction with the floor.

<u>Tips</u>

- Keep your core engaged throughout the exercise to maintain a straight body line.
- Breathe steadily, finding a rhythm with your movements.

Wall Pilates Routine Day 22-25

Warm-up: 2 minutes

1. Wall Plank: 1 minute
2. Plank to Wall Tap: 1 minute
3. Wall Bird Dog: 30 seconds on each side
4. Wall-Assisted Bicycle: 1 minute
5. Wall Scissors: 1 minute
6. Boomerang: 1 minute
7. Neck Pull with Wall Touch: 1 minute
8. Wall Mountain Climbers: 1 minute

Lifestyle Tips to Enhance Your Wall Pilates Workouts

Health and fitness aren't only about working out consistently and eating a nutritious diet. Small, consistent changes to your daily habits can help accelerate your health and well-being, allowing you to maximize every minute of your wall Pilates workouts. Let's look at some lifestyle changes and what they can do for you.

- **Begin your day with gratitude:** Before you even get out of bed in the morning, take a few moments to think about three things you're grateful for. It could be something as simple as the warm sunlight streaming through your window, the cozy comfort of your favorite pajamas, or the fact that you get to wake up and do wall Pilates today! Promoting a practice of gratitude has been shown to boost happiness, reduce stress, and even improve physical health.
- **Hydrate, hydrate, hydrate:** We all know that staying hydrated is essential for overall health, but did you know that it can also improve your Pilates practice? When your body is well-hydrated, your muscles are more pliable, your joints are more lubricated, and your mind is more focused—all of which can lead to better performance on the mat and wall. Aim to drink at least 8 to 10 glasses of water throughout the day.
- **Practice mindful eating:** Eating healthy is about so much more than just choosing the right foods; it's also about how you eat them. Make a point to practice mindful eating at least once a day, whether it's savoring a delicious meal without distractions or taking a few deep breaths before digging in. Pay attention to your food's flavors, textures, and sensations, and try to eat slowly and without judgment. Not only will this help you feel more satisfied and nourished, but it can also improve digestion and reduce stress.
- **Prioritize sleep:** Getting enough high-quality sleep is essential for physical health, mental clarity, and emotional well-being, and yet so many of us struggle to make it a priority. Aim to get at least 7-9 hours of sleep every night, and create a relaxing bedtime routine that helps you wind down and prepare for restful slumber. This might include taking a warm bath, reading a book, or stretching gently.
- **Practice self-compassion:** Nobody's perfect, including you (and me!) There will be days when you don't feel like doing your wall Pilates workout, when you indulge in a less-than-healthy meal, or when you simply don't have the energy to tackle your to-do list. And that's okay.

Instead of beating yourself up or getting caught in a cycle of negative self-talk, practice self-compassion and treat yourself with the same kindness and understanding you would offer a good friend. Remember, progress is more important than perfection, and you're doing your best with what you have.

- **Unplug from technology**: In our hyper-connected world, it's easy to get caught up in the constant buzz of notifications, emails, and social media feeds. However, taking regular breaks from technology is essential for mental clarity, emotional well-being, and an overall sense of presence and connection. Choose a specific time each day to unplug from your devices (like during meals, before bed, or even during your wall Pilates workouts) and focus on the people and experiences right in front of you.

While small, these lifestyle changes can significantly impact your fitness, health, and well-being. Start small, be consistent, and you will begin reaping the rewards for your effort.

Day 26 to 28: Wall Pilates Workouts

Lateral Lunge

This exercise targets the thighs, glutes, and quadriceps while improving lateral stability.

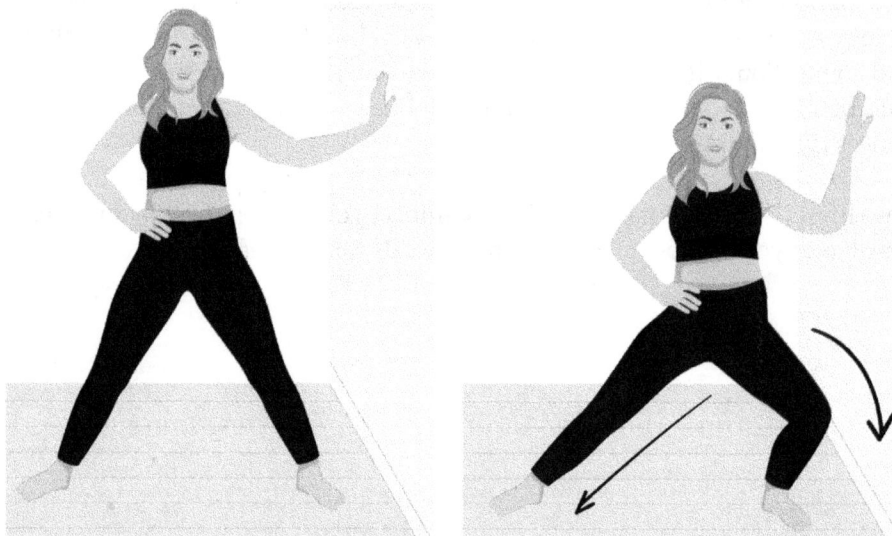

Instructions:

- Stand with your left side facing the wall, about an arm's length away.
- Place your left hand on the wall for balance and support.
- Take a big step to the right with your right foot, about 2–3 feet away.
- Bend your left knee and push your hips back, lowering your body as if sitting back in a chair until your left knee makes contact with the wall. Bend your elbow to facilitate the movement.
- Straighten your right leg, keeping your foot facing forward.
- Hold for 30 seconds.
- Push off with your left foot to return to the starting position.
- Turn around so that your right side faces the wall, and repeat on the other side for 30 seconds.

Modifications:

- Easier: Reduce the depth of the lunge or take a smaller step out.
- Harder: Hold dumbbells in each hand or perform a pulse at the bottom of the lunge.
- Props: Use a yoga mat for better grip if performing on a slippery floor.

Tips:

- Keep your chest up and core engaged throughout the movement.
- Ensure your knee doesn't extend past your toes in the lunge position.
- Keep your weight on the heel of the lunging leg to engage your glutes more.

Wall Figure Four

Wall Figure Four stretches the glutes, piriformis, and outer hip muscles while improving balance and hip mobility.

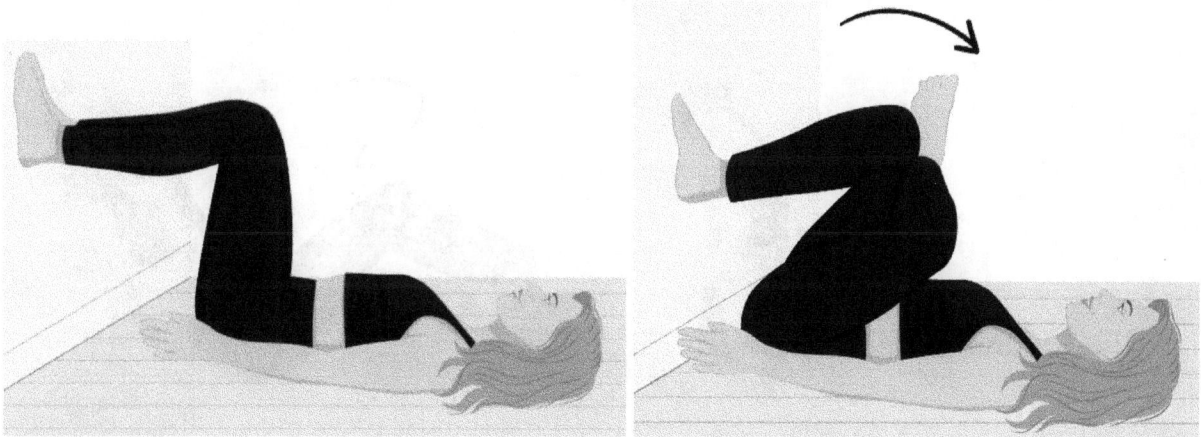

Instructions

- Lie on your back on the floor with your buttocks against the wall, your knees bent, and your feet flat on the wall at about hip-width apart.
- Scoot your hips as close to the wall as possible, keeping your lower back flat on the ground.
- Lift your left foot off the wall and cross your left ankle over your right thigh, just above the knee.
- Your left leg should form a "4" shape against the wall.
- Gently press your left knee away from your body to deepen the stretch.
- Hold this position for 30 seconds.
- Uncross your legs and return both feet to the wall.
- Repeat on the other side, crossing your right ankle over your left thigh for 30 seconds.

Modifications

- Easier: Position yourself further from the wall to decrease the intensity of the stretch.
- Harder: Gently push your foot into the wall to increase the stretch in your opposite hip.
- Props: Place a folded towel or small pillow under your head for neck support if needed.

Tips

- Keep your lower back pressed into the floor throughout the exercise.
- Move your hips slightly away from the wall if the stretch is too intense.

Wall Sit with Ab Twist

This exercise combines the lower body endurance challenge of a wall sit with core rotation, targeting the quadriceps, glutes, and obliques.

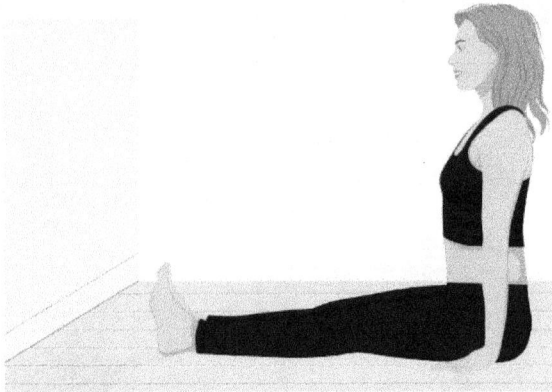

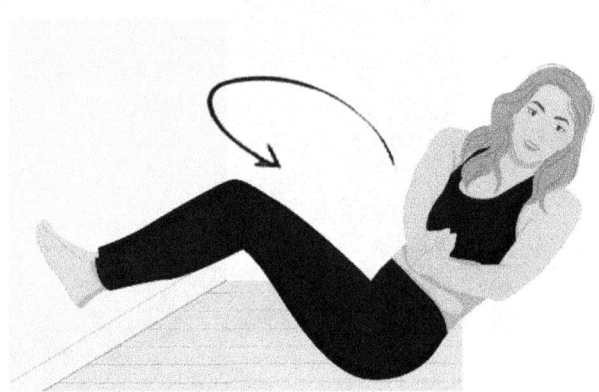

Instructions:

- Start with your feet against the wall, shoulder-width apart, and your buttocks about 2 feet away from the wall.
- Bend your knees and slowly raise your upper body off the floor.
- Bring your hands to your chest, bending your elbows slightly.
- Rotate your upper body to the left first and then the right.
- Continue alternating sides for 1 minute.

Modifications:

- Easier: Hold the wall and sit higher, not going into a full 90-degree angle with your knees.
- Harder: Hold light dumbbells or a medicine ball as you perform the twists.
- Props: Place a small exercise ball between your back and the wall for comfort and feedback.

Tips:

- Keep your core engaged throughout the exercise to support your lower back.
- Breathe steadily: exhale as you twist, inhale as you return to the center.
- Keep your shoulders and head in contact with the wall throughout the movement.
- Focus on rotating from your core, not just moving your arms.
- If you experience knee pain, try adjusting your foot position or reducing the depth of the sit.

Supine Clamshell

This exercise targets the gluteus medius and minimus, crucial for hip stability and proper gait.

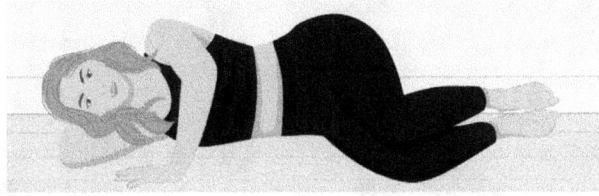

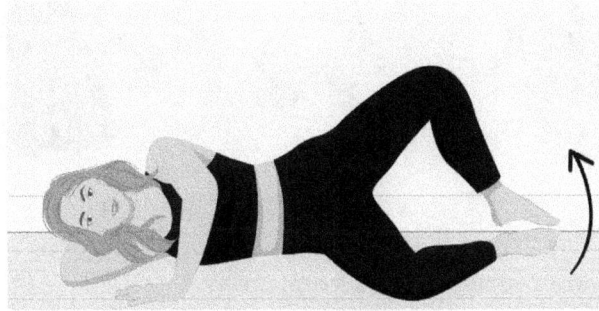

Instructions:

- Lie on your side on the floor with your arm behind your head and your other hand on the ground in front of you.
- Bend your knees at a 90-degree angle, keeping your feet aligned with your back.
- Keep your feet together and lift your top knee towards the ceiling, like a clamshell opening.
- Lift as high as you can before returning to your starting position.
- Repeat for 30 seconds.
- Turn over onto your other side and repeat the exercise for 30 seconds.

Modifications:

- Easier: Reduce the range of motion, not lifting your knee as high.
- Harder: Place a resistance band around your thighs just above the knees.
- Props: Use a yoga mat for comfort on hard floors and a pillow for head support if needed.

Tips:

- Keep your movements slow and controlled throughout the exercise.
- Breathe steadily: exhale as you lift your knee, inhale as you lower it.
- Maintain contact between your back and the wall throughout the movement.
- Focus on initiating the movement from your hip, not rotating your pelvis.
- Keep your feet together throughout the exercise.

Leaning Hip Circles

This exercise improves core strength, spinal mobility, and hip flexibility.

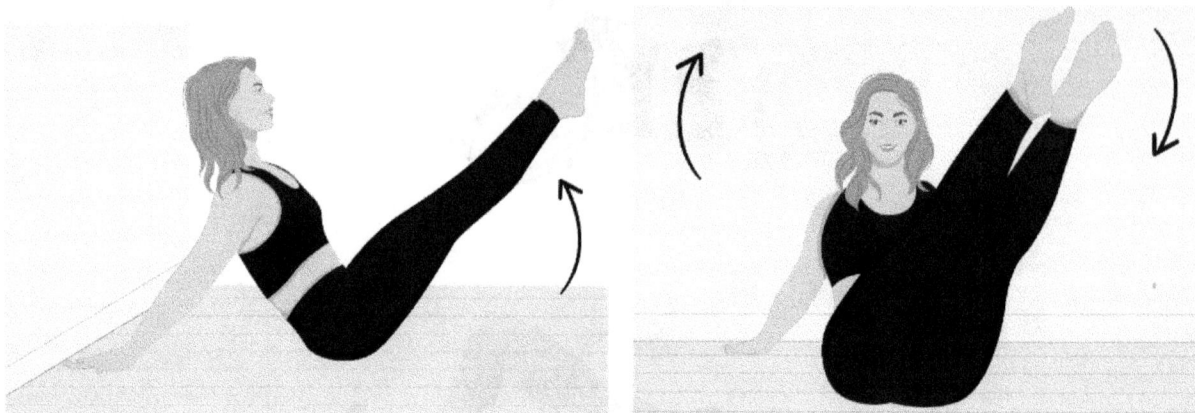

<u>Instructions:</u>

- Sit with your back to the wall about an arm's length away.
- Bend your knees and place your hands behind you so that your fingertips touch the wall's baseboard.
- Use the wall as support by making contact with your shoulders if you would like.
- Engage your core and lift both legs off the floor, straightening them if possible.
- Slowly rotate your legs in a clockwise motion for 30 seconds.
- Place your feet back on the mat to recenter yourself.
- When you are ready, lift both legs off the floor once more and rotate them counterclockwise for 30 seconds.

<u>Modifications:</u>

- Easier: Reduce the range of motion in the twist, or keep both hands on the wall and rotate your torso.
- Harder: Lift the foot farthest from the wall off the ground as you twist, balancing on one leg.
- Props: If you have difficulty reaching the wall comfortably, put a yoga block between your hand and the wall.

<u>Tips:</u>

- Keep your supporting arm slightly bent to avoid locking the elbow.
- Breathe steadily: inhale as you prepare, exhale as you twist, and inhale to return.
- Maintain a stable lower body; the rotation should come from your spine and core.
- Keep your hips facing forward throughout the movement.
- If you feel any strain in your lower back, reduce the range of motion or stop the exercise.

Glute Bridge With Kick

This exercise targets the glutes, hamstrings, and core while improving hip mobility and stability.

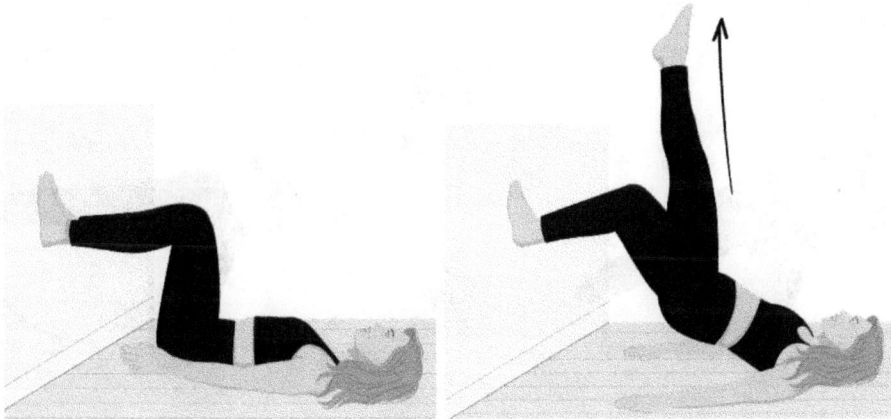

Instructions:

- Lie on your back with buttocks facing the wall and your feet against the wall, knee bent at about 90 degrees.
- Extend your other leg up toward the ceiling, and as you do, lift your buttocks off the ground.
- Place your arms at your sides, palms down, for stability.
- Raise your hips until your body forms a straight line from your shoulders to your knees.
- Keep your leg raised as you lower your buttocks down slightly and immediately thrust back up.
- Continue this movement for 30 seconds.
- Lower your hips back to the starting position.
- Switch legs and repeat the exercise for 30 seconds.

Modifications:

- Easier: Perform the glute bridge without the leg kick.
- Harder: Hold light ankle weights on the kicking leg.
- Props: Use a yoga mat for comfort on hard floors.

Tips:

- Keep your movements controlled throughout the exercise.
- Breathe steadily: exhale as you lift into the bridge, kick, and inhale as you lower your leg.
- Maintain a stable bridge position throughout the leg kicks.
- Press your foot firmly against the wall to help maintain your bridge position.
- Focus on engaging your glutes to lift your hips, not your lower back.

Kneeling Side Kick

This exercise targets the outer thighs, hips, and obliques while improving balance and core stability.

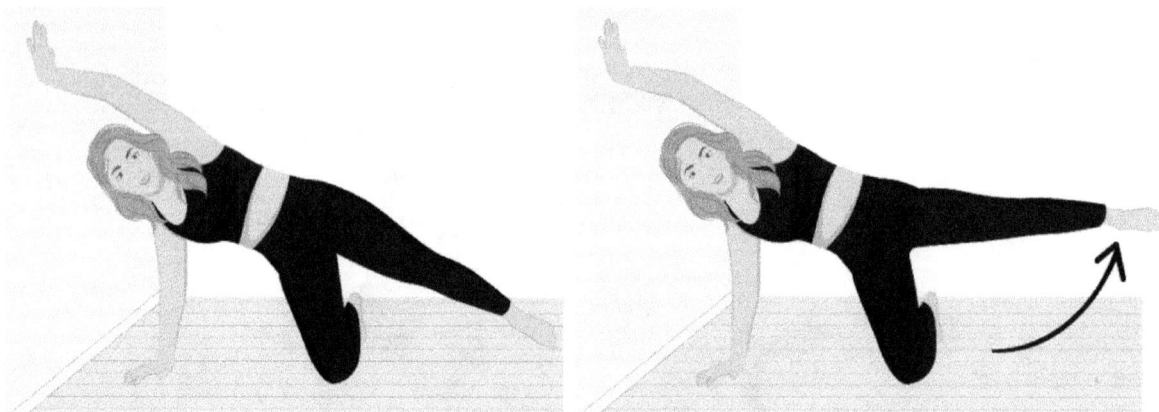

Instructions:

- Start by kneeling on the floor, with the top of your head very close to the wall (almost touching).
- Inhale and lift your left leg straight out to the side. As you do, extend your left arm up and over your head, resting the palm of your hand on the wall.
- Keep your left foot flexed and your body straight from your head to your knees.
- Slowly kick your outer leg up towards the ceiling, keeping it straight.
- Begin to slowly pulse your lifted leg up and down for 30 seconds.
- Place your left leg and hand on the floor and repeat the exercise on the other side for 30 seconds.

Modifications:

- Easier: Reduce the height of the kick or allow your foot to touch the ground between repetitions.
- Harder: Hold the leg up longer at the top of the kick or add small pulses.
- Props: Use a yoga mat or folded towel under your supporting knee for comfort.

Tips:

- Keep your movements slow and controlled throughout the exercise.
- Breathe steadily: exhale as you kick up, inhale as you lower your leg.
- Use the wall as a guide to maintain your alignment; keep the top of your head close to it throughout.
- Focus on lifting from your hip, not arching your back.
- Avoid rotating your hips or pelvis as you kick; keep them squared to the floor.

100s

Wall 100s intensely engage the core muscles, particularly the lower abdominals, while using the wall for leg support.

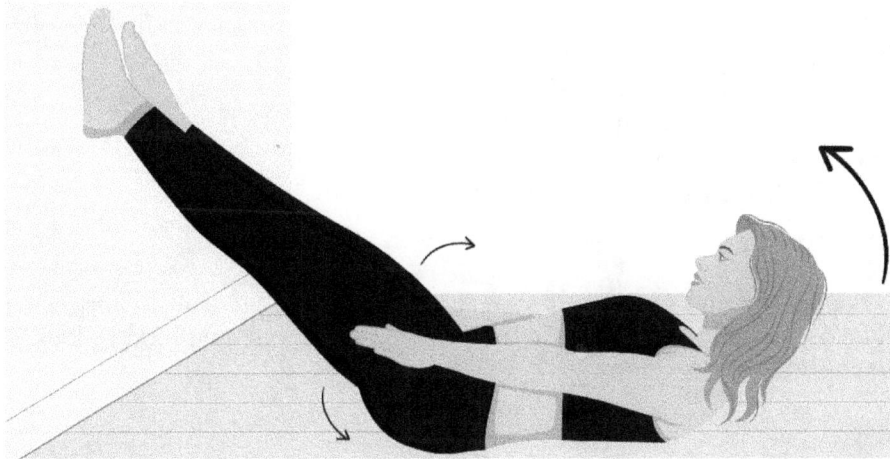

Instructions

- Lie on your back with your legs up the wall, hips close to the baseboard, and your legs straight up the wall.
- Lift your head, neck, and shoulders slightly off the floor, pressing your back into the ground.
- Extend your arms alongside your body, hovering a few inches off the floor, palms down.
- Engage your core by pulling your navel towards your spine.
- Begin pulsing your arms up and down about 2-3 inches, keeping them straight.
- As you pulse, breathe in for five counts and out for five counts.
- Continue this movement and breathing pattern for 1 minute.

Modifications

- Easier: Keep your head on the floor if lifting it causes neck strain, or bend your knees slightly against the wall.
- Harder: Move your hips a few inches away from the wall, maintaining the leg position without wall support.
- Props: Hold light weights or small water bottles in your hands for added upper-body engagement.

Tips

- Keep your core engaged throughout the exercise to protect your lower back.
- Maintain a consistent, controlled pulse with your arms.
- Focus on deep, rhythmic breathing coordinated with your arm movements.
- Keep your shoulders down and away from your ears.

Wall Pilates Routine Day 26-28

Warm-up: 2 minutes

1. Lateral Lunge: 30 seconds on each side
2. Wall Figure Four: 30 seconds on each side
3. Wall Sit With Ab Twist: 30 seconds on each side
4. Supine Clam Shell: 30 seconds on each side
5. Leaning Hip Circles: 30 seconds on each side
6. Glute Bridge With Kick: 30 seconds on each side
7. Kneeling Side Kick: 30 seconds on each side
8. 100s: 1 minute

You have now come to the end of your 28-day structured plan, but wall Pilates is a continuous journey that will help you build a strong, lean body as you grow in strength. Let's look at what you can do to support your wall Pilates journey beyond these 28 days.

CHAPTER 8
YOUR WEIGHT LOSS JOURNEY BEYOND THE 28 DAYS

Congratulations on completing your 28-day challenge. However, this is only the beginning of your wall Pilates journey. Your body has already become stronger and more flexible. Whether you're ready to take on more challenging workouts or want to stick with what you know and repeat the 28-day challenge, that's great.

28 days might not sound like much, but what you've achieved in this time and your dedication have done wonders for your body, even if the scale hasn't moved downward. The number on the scale is not the only measurement of success when it comes to your health and well-being—you've begun to build a strong, lean body, and that is incredible progress.

By making wall Pilates part of your daily routine, you've discovered just how powerful consistency can be. As you move forward from your structured plan, it's important to lay solid foundations for your continued growth—here's how.

- Create your own little wall Pilates haven. It could be a cozy corner in your bedroom or a spot in your office—wherever it feels right. A dedicated space helps you switch off from the world and focus on yourself for those precious minutes.
- Don't be afraid to mix things up. Try different exercises, sequences, or even Pilates styles. Your body and needs are unique, so your practice should be, too. Have fun exploring what feels best for you!
- Set realistic goals that work for you. Remember, your workouts are about practice, not perfection. Some days, you might have time for an extra-long session; others, you might squeeze in a quick 10 minutes, and sometimes life gets in the way completely. That's all okay. The important thing is to show up for yourself with kindness and compassion.
- Keep the big picture in mind. Wall Pilates isn't just about the physical perks. It's about developing deeper awareness, compassion, and resilience in all areas of your life. Approach your practice with curiosity and gratitude for how it supports and changes you.
- Explore some complementary practices. Mindfulness movements like walking meditation, breathwork, or other self-care rituals round out your wellness routine.

- Create your own workouts beyond these 28 days by assembling your own sequence of movements.

Remember, your wall Pilates journey is all about you. Enjoy the process, celebrate your progress, and, most importantly, have fun!

Your Gift

To support you in your wall Pilates health journey, we have put together a *3-in-1 Wall Pilates Journal*. This invaluable tool allows you to keep track of your progress, gain access to daily insights, and plan your meals for your 28 days.

To download your copy of the *3-in-1 Wall Pilates Journal,* scan the QR code or click the URL below.

https://drive.google.com/file/d/1h1lPK1YGvPTO2tmjIIPKC_ho-iCdY_zZ/view?usp=drive_link

Strategies for Maintaining Progress After the Challenge

When you set achievable, measurable targets for yourself, you're laying the groundwork for sustainable success. Progress tracking is also important. Whether you use a fitness app, a journal, or a simple star chart on your fridge, keeping tabs on your journey is a powerful way to stay motivated, accountable, and aware of your incredible progress.

Wall Pilates Prop Guide

Props may be required to deepen your wall Pilates workouts and practice more advanced movements. These small, versatile items can transform your workouts and allow you to complete more advanced movements. In addition, props are excellent for isolating muscles, providing support, or adding challenge to familiar exercises.

Here are some versatile Pilates props you can use, as well as how they can benefit your practice:

Foam Roller: The foam roller is a versatile prop that can enhance balance and challenge your core. Try these exercises:

- Rest your spine on the roller for Arm Circles or Knee Lifts
- Use it horizontally under your pelvis for the Glute Bridge
- Place it beneath your shoulder blades for supine exercises

Hand Weights: In wall Pilates, we use light weights (1-2 pounds) to engage the whole body. They're great for:

- Adding challenge to the Standing Arm Series
- Simulating Reformer exercises like Coordination or Backstroke

Resistance Band: This stretchy band offers both support and resistance:

- Use it for hamstring and lower back stretches
- Add resistance to Side-Lying Leg exercises
- Provide support for Roll Downs or Hip Circles

Tennis Ball: This small, firm ball is excellent for footwork:

- Roll it under your foot while standing or seated
- Use it for gentle massage on tender areas like hips or shoulders

Magic Circle: This classic Pilates prop has many uses:

- Hold it between ankles or thighs to find your midline
- Create instability by balancing on it in side-lying exercises
- Use it for standing balance challenges

Chair: Many Pilates exercises can be modified for a seated position:

- Try forward stretches or spine twists while seated

Yoga Block: This firm foam block is versatile in Pilates:

- Use it as a seat to encourage lengthening your spine

- Place it under your sacrum in the Glute Bridge
- Hold it lightly between hands in a Single Leg Kick to engage back muscles

Incorporating props into your wall Pilates routine can offer new insights into familiar exercises and help you discover more about your body's capabilities. Most of these props are available at local Pilates studios, physical therapy supply stores, or Pilates equipment manufacturers.

Remember, the goal is to enhance your practice, not complicate it. Start with one or two props and gradually explore how they can support your wall Pilates journey. As always, listen to your body and enjoy learning and growing stronger.

CHAPTER 9
BONUS EXERCISES

*T*o deepen your wall Pilates workouts, we've put together a list of bonus exercises that you can incorporate into your routines. These can be added to or replaced by some of the exercises mentioned throughout the book.

Inchworms

Inchworms are a dynamic full-body exercise that improves flexibility in the hamstrings and lower back while strengthening the core, shoulders, and arms.

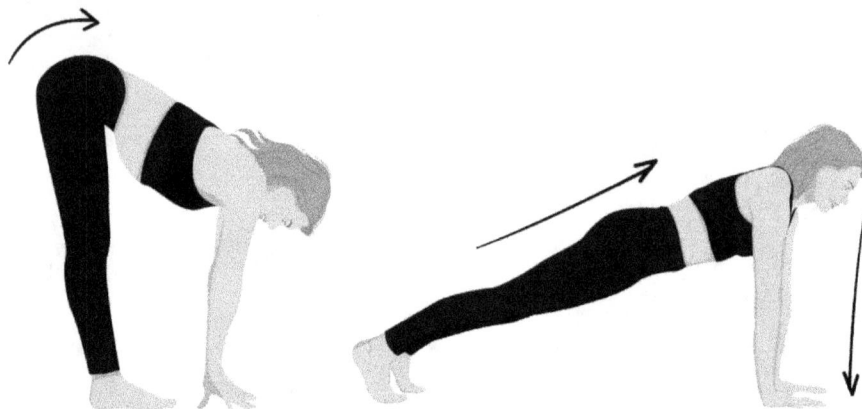

<u>Instructions</u>

- Start by standing tall with your feet hip-width apart.
- Bend at your waist and place your hands on the floor in front of your feet. Bend your knees if needed to reach the floor.
- Walk your hands forward, keeping your legs straight (or slightly bent if necessary) until you're in a high plank position.
- Your body should form a straight line from head to heels.
- Pause briefly in the plank position, engaging your core.
- Now, take tiny steps with your feet, walking them towards your hands while keeping your legs as straight as possible.
- Continue until your feet are as close to your hands as you can comfortably bring them.
- Stand up and return to the starting position.
- Repeat this movement for 1 minute.

<u>Modifications</u>

- Easier: Allow a generous bend in your knees as you walk your hands out and your feet back in.
- Harder: Add a push-up when you're in the plank position or lift one leg off the ground as you hold the plank.
- Props: Use yoga blocks to elevate your hands if you have difficulty reaching the floor.

<u>Tips</u>

- Keep your core engaged throughout the entire movement to protect your lower back.
- Move slowly and with control to maximize the stretch and strength benefits.

Tricep Dips

This exercise primarily targets the triceps muscles at the back of the upper arms while also engaging the chest and shoulders.

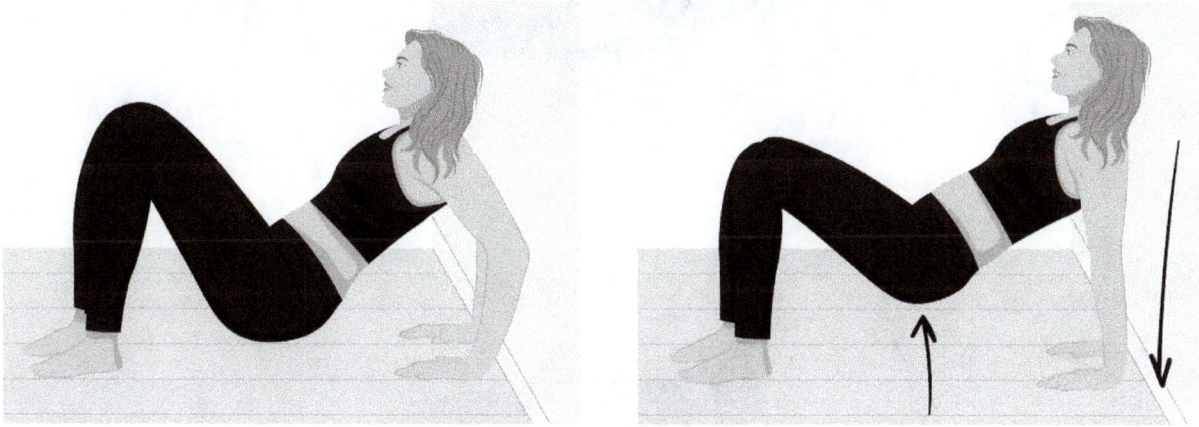

Instructions:

- Sit facing the wall, about arm's length distance.
- Bend your knees and place your feet flat on the floor with your toes touching the wall.
- Bring your hands down to your sides about two hands-lengths away from your buttocks, finger facing forward.
- Lean back and bend your elbows, slowly lowering your body to the mat.
- Push through your palms to straighten your arms, raising your body back up.
- Keep your core engaged and your body close to the wall throughout the movement.
- Repeat for 1 minute.

Modifications:

- Easier: Keep your feet closer to the wall to reduce the load on your arms.
- Harder: Move your feet further from the wall or lift one foot off the ground.
- Props: Use a non-slip mat under your feet if the floor is slippery.

Tips:

- Keep your movements slow and controlled throughout the exercise.
- Breathe steadily: inhale as you lower, exhale as you push up.
- Keep your shoulders down and away from your ears.
- Maintain a slight bend in your elbows at the top of the movement to keep tension on the triceps.
- Keep your core engaged to maintain stability throughout the exercise.

Single Leg Kick

This exercise targets the hamstrings, glutes, and lower back while improving core stability.

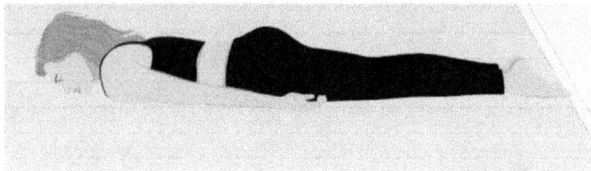

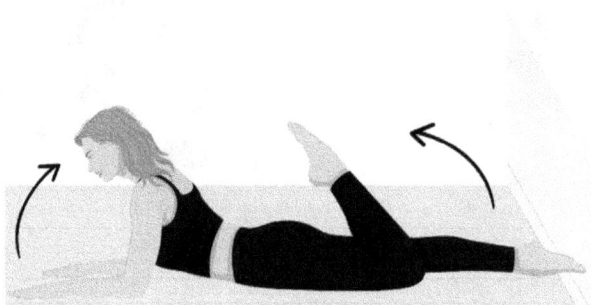

Instructions:

- Lie face down on the floor with your feet pointing toward the wall so you can just touch with your toes pointed. This will keep you aligned.
- Place your forehead on your hands, elbows out to the sides.
- Engage your core and slightly lift your upper body off the floor.
- Bend your right knee, bringing your heel towards your buttocks.
- Kick your right foot towards the wall, aiming to tap it lightly.
- Immediately bend your knee again, bringing your heel back towards your buttocks.
- Perform two quick kicks in succession.
- Lower your right leg and repeat with your left leg.
- Continue alternating legs for 1 minute.

Modifications:

- Easier: Keep your upper body on the floor if lifting causes discomfort.
- Harder: Increase the speed of the kicks or hold your upper body higher off the floor.
- Props: Place a folded towel under your hips for support if needed.

Tips:

- Keep your movements controlled and rhythmic throughout the exercise.
- Breathe steadily: exhale as you kick, inhale as you return.
- Maintain contact between your hips and the floor throughout the movement.
- Focus on using your hamstrings and glutes to power the kicks.

Seated Toe-Touch

This exercise targets the hamstrings, lower back, and calf muscles while improving flexibility and posture.

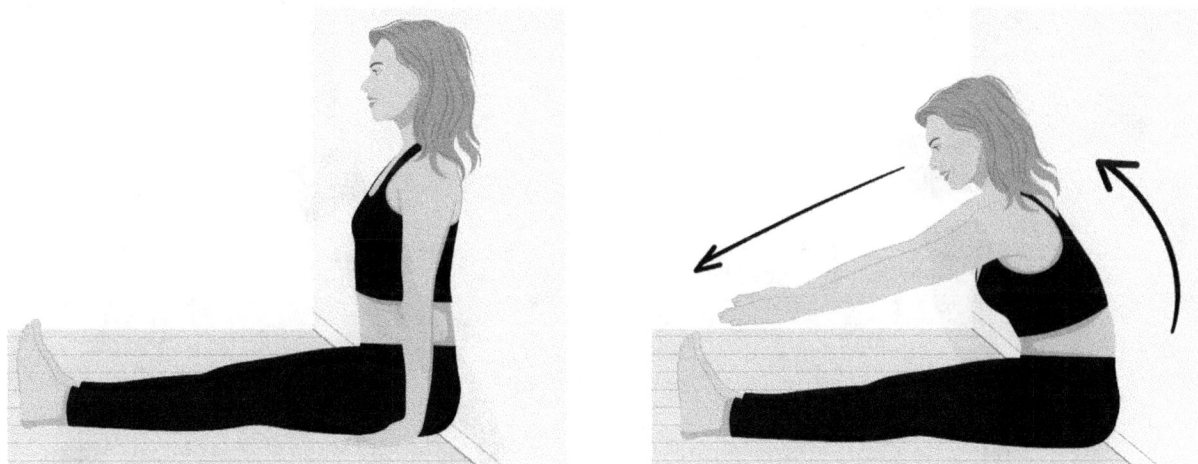

Instructions:

- Sit on the floor with your back against a wall, legs extended straight in front of you.
- Ensure your entire back, from tailbone to head, is in contact with the wall.
- Flex your feet, pointing your toes towards the ceiling.
- Take a deep breath in, lengthening your spine.
- As you exhale, slowly hinge forward at your hips, reaching your hands towards your toes.
- Keep your straight as you fold forward.
- Reach as far as you comfortably can, aiming to touch your toes or ankles.
- Hold the stretch for 1 minute, breathing deeply.
- Slowly roll back up to the starting position.

Modifications:

- Easier: Bend your knees slightly if you can't reach your toes with straight legs.
- Harder: Try to grasp your toes and gently pull yourself further into the stretch.
- Props: Use a yoga strap around your feet if you can't reach your toes.

Tips:

- Keep your movements slow and controlled throughout the exercise.
- Breathe steadily: inhale as you prepare, exhale as you fold forward.
- Maintain contact between your entire back and the wall throughout the movement.
- Focus on hinging at the hips rather than rounding your back.
- If you feel any sharp pain, especially in your lower back, ease out of the stretch.

Push and Pull

This exercise targets the chest, shoulders, upper back, and core muscles.

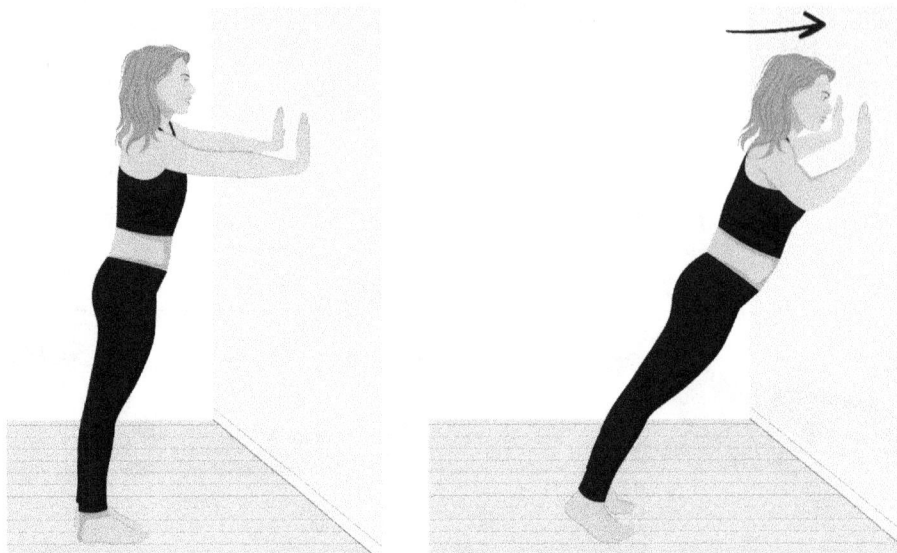

Instructions:

- Stand facing the wall, about an arm's length away.
- Place your palms flat against the wall at shoulder height, slightly wider than shoulder-width apart, in a wider position than push-ups or shoulder presses.
- Step back slightly, leaning into the wall with straight arms.
- Engage your core and keep your body in a straight line from head to heels.
- Begin the "push" phase by slowly bending your elbows to bring your chest towards the wall, as if doing a standing push-up.
- Once your chest is close to the wall, begin the "pull" phase. Try to pull the wall towards you.
- Engage your back muscles and bend your elbows, and bring your shoulder blades together.
- Hold this "pull" position briefly, then slowly return to the starting position.
- Repeat for 1 minute.

Modifications:

- Easier: Stand closer to the wall to reduce the angle and difficulty.
- Harder: Stand further from the wall to increase the angle and engage more muscle.
- Props: Use a textured yoga mat against the wall for better hand grip if needed.

Tips:

- Breathe steadily: inhale during the "push" phase, exhale during the "pull" phase.
- Maintain a straight line from your head to your heels throughout the movement.
- Focus on the contrast between pushing and pulling sensations in your muscles.

Elevated Scissors

This exercise targets the lower abdominals and hip flexors and improves core strength and stability.

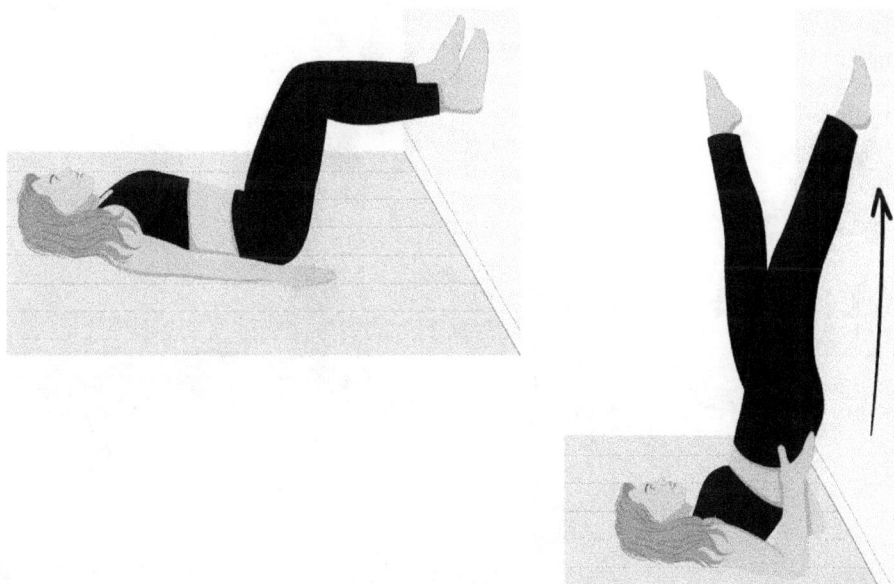

Instructions:

- Lie on your back with your hips close to a wall.
- Extend both legs up the wall, keeping them straight.
- Place your hands on your lower back for stability.
- Engage your core, pressing your upper back into the floor.
- Slowly lift your right leg off the wall, keeping it straight.
- Simultaneously, lift your left leg slightly off the wall.
- Move your legs back and forth in an alternating kicking motion toward your chest, then back to the wall.
- Continue this scissors-like motion for 1 minute.

Modifications:

- Easier: Reduce the range of motion or rest one leg on the wall while the other kicks.
- Harder: Move your legs in a scissor motion without touching the wall, just using it to get into position.
- Props: Use a small pillow under your back for support if needed.

Tips:

- Breathe steadily: exhale as you switch legs, inhale as you prepare for the next switch.
- Maintain contact between your upper back and the floor throughout the movement.
- Focus on using your abdominal muscles to control the leg movements, not momentum.

Corkscrew

This exercise targets the entire core, particularly the obliques, while engaging the hip flexors and improving spinal mobility.

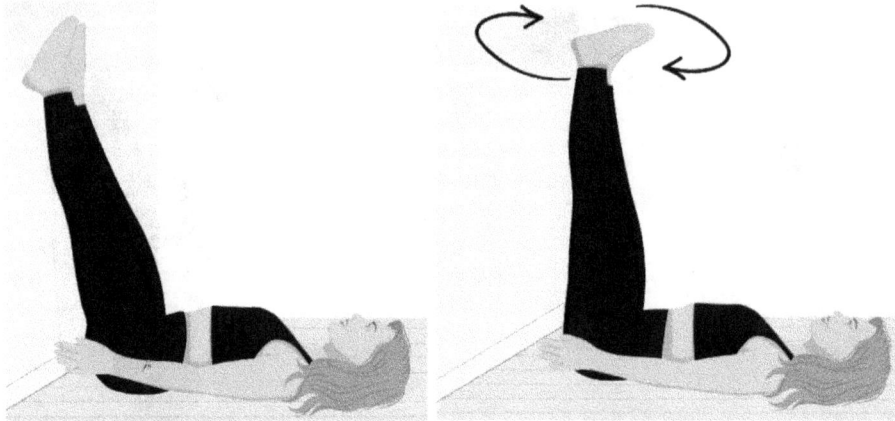

Instructions:

- Lie on your back with your hips close to a wall.
- Extend both legs up the wall, keeping them straight and together.
- Extend your arms out to the sides at shoulder level, palms down for stability.
- Engage your core, pressing your lower back into the floor.
- Keeping your legs straight and together, slowly lower them to the right, creating a diagonal line on the wall.
- Continue the circular motion, bringing your legs down towards your right hip and then across your body towards your left hip.
- Complete the circle by bringing your legs back up to the center of the wall.
- Perform circles in this direction for 30 seconds.
- Reverse the direction and perform circles in the opposite direction for 30 seconds.

Modifications:

- Easier: Reduce the size of the circles or bend your knees slightly.
- Harder: Lift your head and shoulders off the floor, keeping your hands behind your head.
- Props: Use a small pillow under your head for neck support if needed.

Tips:

- Keep your movements slow and controlled throughout the exercise.
- Breathe steadily: inhale as your legs move up, exhale as they move down.
- Maintain contact between your lower back and the floor throughout the movement.
- Focus on using your core muscles to control the leg movements, not momentum.
- Keep your legs together and as straight as possible throughout the exercise.

CONCLUSION

*A*s you come to the end of your wall Pilates journey, take a moment to reflect on how far you've come. From those initial gentle wall exercises to more challenging sequences, you've developed and grown beyond simple movements against a wall. This journey has been about discovering your path to wellness, building strength, adapting to your body's needs, and unlocking your incredible potential for growth and change. With every workout, you've shown that positive transformation is possible and achievable when you commit to yourself.

Wall Pilates has revealed itself as more than just an exercise routine—it's a lifestyle that nurtures body awareness, stability, and self-connection in every movement. Through this practice, you've learned to honor your body's capabilities and limitations, treating it with the care and respect it deserves. You've discovered that true strength and flexibility stem from physical exercise and consistently prioritizing your health with patience, determination, and an open mind.

If you haven't seen all the physical changes you were hoping for yet, don't be discouraged. Fitness is a journey influenced by many factors beyond exercise alone. Celebrate the stronger, more stable body you've cultivated through your practice. Notice how your posture has improved, how you move with more grace and control, and how you're more in tune with your body's needs. These are all significant victories on your path to better health.

Consistency is key. Stick with your wall Pilates routine, gradually increasing the challenge as you feel comfortable. Combine your practice with balanced nutrition, and be patient with yourself. Your body is undergoing positive changes, even if they're not all immediately visible.

As we conclude this journey together, thank you for your dedication and perseverance. Remember, wall Pilates is an ongoing practice, not a destination. There will be progress and setbacks—all part of any fitness journey's natural ebb and flow. Embrace it all with patience and determination, knowing each session moves you forward.

If you've found value in this book, consider sharing your experience with others who might benefit from discovering wall Pilates. Your story could inspire someone else to begin their journey to better health and wellness.

Here's to your continued strength, stability, and well-being through wall Pilates!

RECIPES

*I*n Chapter 2, you were introduced to a meal plan to help fuel your body with the proper nutrition throughout your wall Pilates journey. Below are the complete recipes for this meal plan. Each meal is packed with nutrients and can be mixed and matched to suit your personal tastes, calorie requirements, and budget.

Apple Slices with Almond Butter (Snack)

Serving Size: 1 medium apple with 2 tbsp almond butter

Nutritional Information (approximate):

Calories: 270
Carbohydrates: 28g
Fat: 18g
Sugar: 19g

Ingredients:

- 1 medium apple (about 182g)
- 2 tbsp (32g) almond butter

Directions:

1. Wash the apple thoroughly.
2. Cut the apple into 8 slices, removing the core.
3. Serve with almond butter for dipping.

Avocado Toast with Poached Egg (Breakfast)

Serving Size: 1 slice of toast with toppings

Nutritional Information (approximate):

Calories: 300
Carbohydrates: 20g
Fat: 21g
Sugar: 2g

Ingredients:

- 1 slice whole-grain bread (about 1 oz or 28g)
- 1/2 medium ripe avocado (about 1/4 cup mashed)
- 1 large egg
- 1/4 tsp sea salt
- 1/8 tsp red pepper flakes
- 1 tsp white vinegar (for poaching)
- Water (for poaching)

Directions:

1. Fill a medium saucepan with about 3 inches (7 cm) of water.
2. Add 1 tsp of white vinegar. Bring to a gentle simmer over medium heat.
3. While the water is heating, toast the slice of whole-grain bread to your desired level of crispness.
4. Mash the avocado in a small bowl with a fork until it reaches a spreadable consistency.
5. When the water is simmering, create a gentle whirlpool with a spoon.
6. Crack the egg into a small bowl, then carefully slide it into the center of the whirlpool.
7. Cook for about 3 minutes, or until the white is set but the yolk is still runny.
8. While the egg is poaching, spread the mashed avocado on the toasted bread.
9. Remove the poached egg with a slotted spoon and gently pat dry with a paper towel.
10. Place the poached egg on top of the avocado toast.
11. Sprinkle with sea salt and red pepper flakes.
12. Serve immediately while the toast is still warm and the egg is hot.

My Notes:

_____

_____

Baked Cod with Tomato-Olive Relish (Dinner)

Serving Size: 1 cod filet with relish (approximately 6 oz or 170g)

Nutritional Information (approximate):

Calories: 220
Carbohydrates: 6g
Fat: 10g
Sugar: 2g

Ingredients:

- 6 oz (170g) cod filet
- 1/4 cup (40g) diced tomato
- 2 tbsp (20g) kalamata olives, chopped
- 1 clove garlic, minced
- 1 tbsp fresh parsley, chopped
- 1 tbsp olive oil
- Salt and pepper to taste

Directions:

1. Preheat oven to 400°F (200°C).
2. In a bowl, mix tomato, olives, garlic, parsley, and 1 tsp olive oil.
3. Place cod on a baking sheet lined with parchment paper.
4. Brush cod with remaining olive oil and season with salt and pepper.
5. Top cod with the tomato-olive relish.
6. Bake for 12-15 minutes or until fish flakes easily with a fork.

My Notes:

_____

_____

_____

_____

Blueberry-Almond Smoothie Bowl (Breakfast)

Serving Size: 1 bowl (approximately 2 cups)

Nutritional Information (approximate):

Calories: 380
Carbohydrates: 55g
Fat: 18g
Sugar: 32g

Ingredients:

- 1 cup (150g) frozen blueberries
- 1 ripe banana
- 1 tbsp (16g) almond butter
- 1/2 cup (120ml) unsweetened almond milk
- 1 tbsp (9g) sliced almonds
- 1 tbsp (5g) shredded coconut
- 1 tsp honey

Directions:

1. In a blender, combine frozen blueberries, banana, almond butter, and almond milk.
2. Blend until smooth, adding more almond milk if needed.
3. Pour into a bowl.
4. Top with sliced almonds and shredded coconut.
5. Drizzle honey over the top.
6. Serve immediately.

My Notes:

_____

_____

_____

_____

Breakfast Burrito (Breakfast)

Serving Size: 1 burrito

Nutritional Information (approximate):

Calories: 450
Carbohydrates: 40g
Fat: 25g
Sugar: 3g

Ingredients:

- 2 large eggs
- 1/4 cup (40g) canned black beans, rinsed and drained
- 2 tbsp (30g) salsa
- 2 tbsp (20g) shredded cheddar cheese
- 1 large (10-inch) whole-grain tortilla
- 1/4 avocado, sliced
- Hot sauce to taste (optional)

Directions:

1. In a bowl, whisk the eggs.
2. Heat a non-stick skillet over medium heat.
3. Pour in the eggs and cook, stirring gently, until they begin to set.
4. Add black beans and continue cooking until eggs are scrambled and beans are warm.
5. Stir in salsa and cheese.
6. Warm the tortilla in a separate pan or microwave for 10 seconds.
7. Place the egg mixture in the center of the tortilla.
8. Fold in the sides and roll up tightly.
9. Serve with sliced avocado and hot sauce on the side if desired.

My Notes:

_____

_____

_____

Carrot Sticks and Hummus (Snack)

Serving Size: 1 cup carrot sticks with 2 tbsp hummus

Nutritional Information (approximate):

Calories: 100
Carbohydrates: 14g
Fat: 5g
Sugar: 6g

Ingredients:

- 1 cup (128g) carrot sticks (about 2 medium carrots)
- 2 tbsp (30g) hummus

Directions:

1. Wash and peel the carrots.
2. Cut the carrots into sticks about 3 inches long and 1/2 inch wide.
3. Serve with hummus for dipping.

My Notes:

_____

_____

_____

_____

_____

Caprese Salad with Grilled Chicken (Lunch)

Serving Size: 1 salad

Nutritional Information (approximate):

Calories: 380
Carbohydrates: 10g
Fat: 22g
Sugar: 6g

Ingredients:

- 2 cups (60g) mixed salad greens
- 4 oz (115g) grilled chicken breast, sliced
- 2 oz (60g) fresh mozzarella, sliced
- 1 medium tomato, sliced
- 5-6 fresh basil leaves
- 1 tbsp (15ml) balsamic vinaigrette
- Salt and pepper to taste

Directions:

1. Arrange mixed greens on a plate.
2. Top with sliced grilled chicken, mozzarella, and tomato.
3. Tear basil leaves and sprinkle over the salad.
4. Drizzle with balsamic vinaigrette.
5. Season with salt and pepper to taste.
6. Serve immediately.

My Notes:

_____

_____

_____

_____

Celery Sticks with Peanut Butter and Raisins (Snack)

Serving Size: 3 celery sticks

Nutritional Information (approximate):

Calories: 150
Carbohydrates: 11g
Fat: 11g
Sugar: 7g

Ingredients:

- 3 celery sticks (about 5 inches long each)
- 2 tbsp (32g) peanut butter
- 1 tbsp (15g) raisins

Directions:

1. Wash and cut celery into 5-inch sticks.
2. Fill each celery stick with peanut butter.
3. Sprinkle raisins over the peanut butter.
4. Serve immediately or refrigerate for up to 24 hours.

My Notes:

_____

_____

_____

_____

_____

Cherry Tomatoes with Mozzarella and Basil (Snack)

Serving Size: 1 cup (about 10-12 pieces)

Nutritional Information (approximate):

Calories: 150
Carbohydrates: 5g
Fat: 11g
Sugar: 3g

Ingredients:

- 1 cup (150g) cherry tomatoes
- 1/2 cup (60g) small mozzarella balls (ciliegine)
- 10-12 fresh basil leaves
- 1 tsp olive oil
- Salt and pepper to taste

Directions:

1. Wash and halve the cherry tomatoes.
2. Cut mozzarella balls in half if they're larger than the tomatoes.
3. Thread a tomato half, a basil leaf, and a mozzarella half onto a toothpick.
4. Arrange on a plate, drizzle with olive oil, and sprinkle with salt and pepper.
5. Serve immediately or refrigerate for up to 2 hours.

My Notes:

_____

_____

_____

_____

Chia Seed Pudding with Mango (Breakfast)

Serving Size: 1 jar (approximately 1 cup)

Nutritional Information (approximate):

Calories: 300
Carbohydrates: 35g
Fat: 18g
Sugar: 20g

Ingredients:

- 3 tbsp (45g) chia seeds
- 1 cup (240ml) coconut milk
- 1 tsp honey
- 1/2 cup (80g) diced mango
- 1 tbsp (5g) shredded coconut

Directions:

1. In a jar, whisk together chia seeds, coconut milk, and honey.
2. Cover and refrigerate overnight or for at least 4 hours.
3. In the morning, stir the pudding and top with diced mango.
4. Sprinkle shredded coconut over the top.
5. Serve chilled.

My Notes:

_____

_____

_____

_____

Chocolate-Banana Protein Pancakes (Breakfast)

Serving Size: 3 pancakes

Nutritional Information (approximate):

Calories: 380
Carbohydrates: 45g
Fat: 14g
Sugar: 18g

Ingredients:

- 1 ripe banana
- 2 large eggs
- 1 scoop (30g) chocolate protein powder
- 1 tbsp (5g) cocoa powder
- 1/4 tsp baking powder
- 1 tbsp (16g) almond butter for topping
- 1/2 banana, sliced for topping

Directions:

1. In a blender, combine banana, eggs, protein powder, cocoa powder, and baking powder. Blend until smooth.
2. Heat a non-stick skillet over medium heat.
3. Pour about 1/4 cup of batter for each pancake.
4. Cook for 2-3 minutes until bubbles form on top, then flip and cook for another 1-2 minutes.
5. Repeat with remaining batter.
6. Serve pancakes topped with a drizzle of almond butter and sliced banana.

My Notes:

_____

_____

_____

_____

Cucumber Slices with Cream Cheese and Smoked Salmon (Snack)

Serving Size: 6 slices

Nutritional Information (approximate):

Calories: 120
Carbohydrates: 4g
Fat: 8g
Sugar: 2g

Ingredients:

- 1/2 medium cucumber (about 100g)
- 2 tbsp (30g) cream cheese
- 2 oz (60g) smoked salmon
- Fresh dill for garnish (optional)

Directions:

1. Wash and slice cucumber into 6 rounds, about 1/4 inch thick.
2. Spread cream cheese evenly on each cucumber slice.
3. Top each slice with a small piece of smoked salmon.
4. Garnish with fresh dill if desired.
5. Serve immediately.

My Notes:

_____

_____

_____

_____

Curried Chicken Salad (Lunch)

Serving Size: 1 cup

Nutritional Information (approximate):

Calories: 280
Carbohydrates: 12g
Fat: 14g
Sugar: 8g

Ingredients:

- 1 cup (140g) cooked chicken breast, shredded
- 2 tbsp (30g) Greek yogurt
- 1 tsp curry powder
- 1/4 cup (30g) apple, diced
- 1 tbsp fresh cilantro, chopped
- Salt and pepper to taste
- Optional: 1 whole-grain pita or 1 cup mixed greens for serving

Directions:

1. In a bowl, mix Greek yogurt and curry powder.
2. Add shredded chicken, diced apple, and chopped cilantro. Mix well.
3. Season with salt and pepper to taste.
4. Serve over mixed greens or in a whole-grain pita.
5. Refrigerate any leftovers in an airtight container for up to 2 days.

My Notes:

_____

_____

_____

_____

_____

Egg and Veggie Muffins (Breakfast)

Serving Size: 2 muffins

Nutritional Information (approximate):

Calories: 180
Carbohydrates: 4g
Fat: 13g
Sugar: 2g

Ingredients:

- 6 large eggs
- 1/4 cup (40g) diced bell pepper
- 1/2 cup (15g) fresh spinach, chopped
- 1/4 cup (28g) shredded cheese (cheddar or mozzarella)
- Salt and pepper to taste
- Cooking spray

Directions:

1. Preheat oven to 350°F (175°C).
2. In a large bowl, whisk eggs with salt and pepper.
3. Stir in diced bell pepper, chopped spinach, and shredded cheese.
4. Grease a 6-cup muffin tin with cooking spray.
5. Divide egg mixture evenly among the muffin cups.
6. Bake for 20-25 minutes, until eggs are set and slightly golden on top.
7. Let cool for 5 minutes before removing from the tin.
8. Serve warm or at room temperature.
9. Store leftovers in an airtight container in the refrigerator for up to 3 days.

My Notes:

_____

_____

_____

_____

Greek Yogurt Parfait (Breakfast)

Serving Size: 1 parfait (approximately 12 oz or 340g)

Nutritional Information (approximate):

Calories: 320
Carbohydrates: 40g
Fat: 12g
Sugar: 25g

Ingredients:

- 1 cup (240g) plain Greek yogurt
- 1/4 cup (30g) homemade granola
- 1/2 cup (75g) mixed fresh berries (strawberries, blueberries, raspberries)
- 1 tsp maple syrup

Directions:

1. In a 12 oz (340g) jar or glass, start with a layer of 1/3 cup Greek yogurt.
2. Add 2 tablespoons of mixed berries on top of the yogurt.
3. Sprinkle 2 tablespoons of granola over the berries.
4. Repeat the layering process once more.
5. Top with the remaining Greek yogurt.
6. Finish with the remaining berries and granola on top.
7. Drizzle 1 teaspoon of maple syrup over the parfait.
8. Serve immediately, or refrigerate for up to 2 hours before serving.

My Notes:

_____

_____

_____

_____

Greek Salad with Grilled Shrimp (Lunch)

Serving Size: 1 large salad (approximately 3 cups or 300g)

Nutritional Information (approximate):

Calories: 380
Carbohydrates: 20g
Fat: 25g
Sugar: 8g

Ingredients:

- 2 cups (60g) mixed greens
- 1/4 cup (30g) cucumber, diced
- 1/4 cup (40g) tomato, diced
- 2 tbsp (20g) red onion, thinly sliced
- 2 tbsp (20g) kalamata olives, pitted
- 2 tbsp (30g) feta cheese, crumbled
- 4 oz (115g) grilled shrimp
- 1 tsp fresh dill, chopped

For the dressing:

- 1 tbsp olive oil
- 1 tbsp lemon juice
- 1/4 tsp dried oregano
- Salt and pepper to taste

Directions:

1. In a large bowl, combine mixed greens, cucumber, tomato, red onion, olives, and feta cheese.
2. Whisk together olive oil, lemon juice, oregano, salt, and pepper for the dressing.
3. Toss the salad with the dressing.
4. Top with grilled shrimp and sprinkle with fresh dill.
5. Serve immediately.

My Notes:

_____

_____

Greek Yogurt with Honey and Walnuts (Snack)

Serving Size: 1 cup

Nutritional Information (approximate):

Calories: 220
Carbohydrates: 25g
Fat: 10g
Sugar: 22g

Ingredients:

- 1 cup (245g) plain Greek yogurt
- 1 tbsp (21g) honey
- 1 tbsp (7g) chopped walnuts

Directions:

1. Spoon Greek yogurt into a bowl.
2. Drizzle honey over the yogurt.
3. Sprinkle chopped walnuts on top.
4. Serve immediately.

My Notes:

_____

_____

_____

_____

_____

Grilled Salmon with Asparagus (Dinner)

Serving Size: 1 salmon filet with asparagus and sauce

Nutritional Information (approximate):

Calories: 380
Carbohydrates: 8g
Fat: 25g
Sugar: 3g

Ingredients:

- 1 (6 oz / 170g) salmon filet
- 8 asparagus spears, trimmed
- 1 tbsp (15ml) olive oil
- 1 lemon, half juiced and half sliced
- 1 clove garlic, minced
- 1 tsp dried herbs (mix of dill, thyme, and parsley)
- Salt and pepper to taste

For the yogurt-dill sauce:

- 2 tbsp (30g) Greek yogurt
- 1 tsp fresh dill, chopped
- 1/2 tsp lemon juice
- Salt and pepper to taste

Directions:

1. Preheat grill to medium-high heat (about 400°F / 200°C).
2. In a small bowl, mix olive oil, lemon juice, minced garlic, and dried herbs.
3. Brush the salmon and asparagus with the herb mixture. Season with salt and pepper.
4. Place salmon skin-side down on the grill. Arrange lemon slices on top.
5. Grill salmon for 4-5 minutes, then add asparagus to the grill.
6. Cook for an additional 3-4 minutes, or until salmon is flaky and asparagus is tender-crisp.
7. While the salmon cooks, mix Greek yogurt, chopped dill, lemon juice, salt, and pepper in a small bowl.
8. Remove salmon and asparagus from the grill.
9. Serve the salmon with asparagus on the side and a dollop of yogurt-dill sauce.

My Notes:

Grilled Steak with Chimichurri (Dinner)

Serving Size: 4 oz steak with 2 tbsp chimichurri

Nutritional Information (approximate):

Calories: 320
Carbohydrates: 2g
Fat: 24g
Sugar: 0g

Ingredients:

- 4 oz (115g) flank steak
- Salt and pepper to taste

For the chimichurri:

- 1/4 cup (15g) fresh parsley, finely chopped
- 1 garlic clove, minced
- 1 tbsp red wine vinegar
- 2 tbsp olive oil
- 1/4 tsp red pepper flakes
- Salt to taste

Directions:

1. Season steak with salt and pepper.
2. Preheat grill to medium-high heat.
3. Grill steak for 4-5 minutes per side for medium-rare.
4. While steak is cooking, mix all chimichurri ingredients in a bowl.
5. Let steak rest for 5 minutes, then slice thinly against the grain.
6. Serve steak with chimichurri sauce on top.

My Notes:

_____

_____

_____

Hard-Boiled Eggs with Everything Bagel Seasoning (Snack)

Serving Size: 2 eggs

Nutritional Information (approximate):

Calories: 160
Carbohydrates: 1g
Fat: 11g
Sugar: 0g

Ingredients:

- 2 large eggs
- 1 tsp everything bagel seasoning

Directions:

1. Place eggs in a saucepan and cover with 1 inch (3cm) of cold water.
2. Bring water to a boil over high heat.
3. Remove from heat, cover, and let sit for 9-12 minutes.
4. Transfer eggs to an ice bath to cool for 5 minutes.
5. Peel eggs, cut in half, and sprinkle with everything bagel seasoning.

My Notes:

_____

_____

_____

_____

_____

Harvest Grain Bowl (Lunch)

Serving Size: 1 bowl

Nutritional Information (approximate):

Calories: 450
Carbohydrates: 65g
Fat: 20g
Sugar: 8g

Ingredients:

- 1/2 cup (85g) cooked quinoa or farro
- 1/2 cup (75g) roasted sweet potatoes, cubed
- 1/2 cup (50g) roasted Brussels sprouts, halved
- 1/4 cup (40g) cooked chickpeas
- 1 oz (30g) crumbled feta cheese

For the tahini-lemon dressing:

- 1 tbsp (15g) tahini
- 1 tbsp (15ml) lemon juice
- 1 tsp olive oil
- 1 tsp water
- Salt and pepper to taste

Directions:

1. In a bowl, combine cooked quinoa or farro, roasted sweet potatoes, Brussels sprouts, and chickpeas.
2. In a small bowl, whisk together tahini, lemon juice, olive oil, and water to make the dressing. Season with salt and pepper.
3. Drizzle the dressing over the grain bowl.
4. Top with crumbled feta cheese.
5. Serve at room temperature or slightly warm.

My Notes:

_____

_____

Homemade Hummus with Veggie Sticks (Snack)

Serving Size: 1/4 cup hummus with 1 cup veggie sticks

Nutritional Information (approximate):

Calories: 180
Carbohydrates: 20g
Fat: 10g
Sugar: 5g

Ingredients for Hummus:

- 1 can (15 oz/425g) chickpeas, drained and rinsed
- 2 tbsp tahini
- 2 tbsp lemon juice
- 1 clove garlic, minced
- 2 tbsp olive oil
- 1/4 tsp salt
- 2-3 tbsp water

For Veggie Sticks:

- 1 cup mixed raw vegetables (carrots, celery, bell peppers, cucumber)

Directions:

1. In a food processor, blend chickpeas, tahini, lemon juice, garlic, olive oil, and salt until smooth.
2. Add water gradually to reach desired consistency.
3. Transfer hummus to a serving bowl.
4. Wash and cut vegetables into sticks.
5. Serve hummus with veggie sticks.
6. Store leftover hummus in an airtight container in the refrigerator for up to 5 days.

My Notes:

_____

_____

_____

Homemade Kale Chips (Snack)

Serving Size: 1 cup

Nutritional Information (approximate):

Calories: 110
Carbohydrates: 6g
Fat: 9g
Sugar: 0g

Ingredients:

- 2 cups (67g) fresh kale leaves torn into bite-sized pieces
- 1 tbsp (15ml) olive oil
- 1/4 tsp salt
- Optional: 1/4 tsp garlic powder or other seasonings

Directions:

1. Preheat oven to 300°F (150°C).
2. Wash kale leaves and dry thoroughly.
3. In a large bowl, toss kale with olive oil, salt (and optional seasonings).
4. Spread kale in a single layer on a baking sheet lined with parchment paper.
5. Bake for 10-15 minutes, until edges are slightly brown but not burnt.
6. Let cool for 5 minutes before serving.
7. Store in an airtight container for up to 2 days.

My Notes:

Homemade Trail Mix (Snack)

Serving Size: 1/4 cup (about 30g)

Nutritional Information (approximate):

Calories: 160
Carbohydrates: 12g
Fat: 12g
Sugar: 7g

Ingredients:

- 1/4 cup (35g) raw almonds
- 1/4 cup (30g) raw cashews
- 1/4 cup (30g) pumpkin seeds
- 1/4 cup (40g) dried cranberries
- 1/4 cup (30g) dark chocolate chips (optional)

Directions:

1. In a large bowl, combine all ingredients.
2. Mix well to ensure even distribution.
3. Store in an airtight container at room temperature for up to 2 weeks.
4. Serve 1/4 cup as a single portion.

Note: This recipe makes about 1 1/4 cups of trail mix. Adjust the ingredients based on personal preferences and dietary needs.

My Notes:

_____

_____

_____

_____

_____

Lentil and Vegetable Curry (Dinner)

Serving Size: 1 cup curry with 1/2 cup brown rice

Nutritional Information (approximate):

Calories: 380
Carbohydrates: 65g
Fat: 10g
Sugar: 8g

Ingredients:

- 1/2 cup (100g) red lentils
- 1/2 cup (75g) sweet potato, diced
- 1/2 cup (50g) cauliflower florets
- 1/4 cup (35g) peas
- 1/2 cup (120ml) coconut milk
- 1/2 cup (120ml) vegetable broth
- 1 tbsp curry powder
- 1/2 cup (85g) cooked brown rice
- Salt to taste

Directions:

1. Rinse lentils in cold water.
2. In a pot, combine lentils, sweet potato, cauliflower, peas, coconut milk, broth, and curry powder.
3. Bring to a boil, then reduce heat and simmer for 20-25 minutes until lentils and vegetables are tender.
4. Season with salt to taste.
5. Serve over brown rice.

My Notes:

_____

_____

_____

Mason Jar Cobb Salad (Lunch)

Serving Size: 1 mason jar (16 oz or 475 ml)

Nutritional Information (approximate):

Calories: 400
Carbohydrates: 10g
Fat: 32g
Sugar: 4g

Ingredients:

- 1 cup (50g) chopped romaine lettuce
- 1 hard-boiled egg, chopped
- 1/4 avocado, diced
- 1/4 cup (37g) cherry tomatoes, halved
- 2 tbsp (15g) cooked bacon, crumbled
- 2 tbsp (30g) crumbled blue cheese
- 2 tbsp red wine vinaigrette

Directions:

1. Pour vinaigrette into the bottom of the mason jar.
2. Layer ingredients in the following order: tomatoes, bacon, egg, avocado, blue cheese, and lettuce.
3. Seal jar and refrigerate until ready to eat.
4. To serve, shake jar to distribute dressing, then pour onto a plate or eat directly from the jar.

My Notes:

_____

_____

_____

_____

Mediterranean Quinoa Salad (Lunch)

Serving Size: 1 bowl (approximately 2 cups or 340g)

Nutritional Information (approximate):

Calories: 380
Carbohydrates: 45g
Fat: 20g
Sugar: 5g

Ingredients:

- 1/2 cup (85g) uncooked quinoa
- 1 cup (240ml) water
- 1/2 cup (75g) cherry tomatoes, halved
- 1/4 cup (30g) cucumber, diced
- 2 tbsp (20g) red onion, finely chopped
- 2 tbsp (20g) kalamata olives, pitted and halved
- 2 tbsp (30g) feta cheese, crumbled
- 1 tbsp (15ml) extra virgin olive oil
- 1 tbsp (15ml) lemon juice
- 1/4 tsp dried oregano
- Salt and pepper to taste

Directions:

1. Rinse quinoa in a fine-mesh strainer under cold water.
2. In a medium saucepan, combine quinoa and water. Bring to a boil.
3. Reduce heat to low, cover, and simmer for about 15 minutes or until water is absorbed.
4. Remove from heat and let stand, covered, for 5 minutes. Fluff with a fork and let cool.
5. In a large bowl, combine the cooled quinoa, tomatoes, cucumber, red onion, and olives.
6. In a small bowl, whisk together olive oil, lemon juice, and oregano to make the vinaigrette.
7. Pour the vinaigrette over the quinoa mixture and toss gently to combine.
8. Add the crumbled feta cheese and toss lightly.
9. Season with salt and pepper to taste.
10. Serve immediately or chill in the refrigerator for at least 30 minutes for a refreshing cold salad.

My Notes:

Overnight Oats with Berries (Breakfast)

Serving Size: 1 jar (approximately 1 cup)

Nutritional Information (approximate):

Calories: 350
Carbohydrates: 50g
Fat: 12g
Sugar: 18g

Ingredients:

- 1/2 cup (45g) rolled oats
- 1/2 cup (120ml) unsweetened almond milk
- 1/4 cup (60g) Greek yogurt
- 1 tbsp (15g) chia seeds
- 1 tsp honey
- 1/2 cup (75g) mixed fresh berries
- 1/4 tsp ground cinnamon

Directions:

1. In a jar or container, combine oats, almond milk, Greek yogurt, chia seeds, and honey.
2. Stir well to mix all ingredients.
3. Cover and refrigerate overnight or for at least 6 hours.
4. In the morning, stir the oats and top with fresh berries and a sprinkle of cinnamon.
5. Serve cold or warm gently if preferred.

My Notes:

_____

_____

_____

_____

Peanut Butter Banana Smoothie (Breakfast)

Serving Size: 1 glass (approximately 16 oz or 470ml)

Nutritional Information (approximate):

Calories: 380
Carbohydrates: 45g
Fat: 18g
Sugar: 22g

Ingredients:

- 1 medium frozen banana, sliced
- 2 tbsp (32g) peanut butter
- 1 cup (240ml) unsweetened almond milk
- 1 scoop (30g) vanilla protein powder
- 1/2 cup (120ml) ice

Directions:

1. Add all ingredients to a blender.
2. Blend on high speed until smooth and creamy, about 30-45 seconds.
3. If the smoothie is too thick, add a little more almond milk and blend again.
4. Pour into a glass and serve immediately.

My Notes:

_____

_____

_____

_____

_____

Pesto Chicken Salad (Lunch)

Serving Size: 1 cup chicken salad over 1 cup mixed greens

Nutritional Information (approximate):

Calories: 350
Carbohydrates: 8g
Fat: 25g
Sugar: 2g

Ingredients:

- 1 cup (140g) cooked chicken breast, shredded
- 2 tbsp (30g) homemade or store-bought pesto
- 2 tbsp (20g) celery, diced
- 1 tbsp (10g) sliced almonds
- 1 cup (30g) mixed greens
- Salt and pepper to taste

Directions:

1. In a bowl, mix shredded chicken, pesto, celery, and sliced almonds.
2. Season with salt and pepper to taste.
3. Serve over a bed of mixed greens or in a hollowed-out tomato.
4. If using a tomato, cut the top off and scoop out the seeds and some of the flesh to create a bowl.
5. Fill the tomato with the chicken salad mixture.
6. Serve chilled

My Notes:

_____

_____

_____

_____

Quinoa-Stuffed Bell Peppers (Dinner)

Serving Size: 1 stuffed pepper half

Nutritional Information (approximate):

Calories: 250
Carbohydrates: 40g
Fat: 7g
Sugar: 5g

Ingredients:

- 1 large bell pepper, halved and seeds removed
- 1/2 cup (85g) cooked quinoa
- 1/4 cup (40g) black beans, drained and rinsed
- 1/4 cup (35g) corn kernels
- 2 tbsp salsa
- 2 tbsp (20g) shredded cheese
- Salt and pepper to taste

Directions:

1. Preheat oven to 375°F (190°C).
2. In a bowl, mix quinoa, black beans, corn, salsa, and half the cheese.
3. Season with salt and pepper.
4. Stuff mixture into bell pepper halves.
5. Top with remaining cheese.
6. Place in a baking dish and bake for 25-30 minutes until peppers are tender.

My Notes:

_____

_____

_____

_____

Roasted Chickpeas with Cumin and Smoked Paprika (Snack)

Serving Size: 1/4 cup (about 30g)

Nutritional Information (approximate):

Calories: 120
Carbohydrates: 18g
Fat: 4g
Sugar: 3g

Ingredients:

- 1 can (15 oz/425g) chickpeas, drained and rinsed
- 1 tbsp olive oil
- 1/2 tsp ground cumin
- 1/2 tsp smoked paprika
- 1/4 tsp salt

Directions:

1. Preheat oven to 400°F (200°C).
2. Pat chickpeas dry with a paper towel.
3. In a bowl, toss chickpeas with olive oil, cumin, smoked paprika, and salt.
4. Spread chickpeas on a baking sheet in a single layer.
5. Roast for 20-30 minutes, shaking the pan halfway through, until chickpeas are crispy.
6. Let cool for 5 minutes before serving.
7. Store in an airtight container at room temperature for up to 3 days.

My Notes:

_____

_____

_____

_____

Savory Breakfast Bowl (Breakfast)

Serving Size: 1 bowl (approximately 2 cups or 400-450g total)

Nutritional Information (approximate):

Calories: 350
Carbohydrates: 30g
Fat: 22g
Sugar: 5g

Ingredients:

- 1 cup (67g) chopped kale
- 1/2 cup (75g) diced sweet potato
- 1 large egg
- 1/4 avocado, sliced
- 2 tbsp (30g) salsa
- 1 tsp olive oil
- Salt and pepper to taste

Directions:

1. Preheat oven to 400°F (200°C).
2. Toss sweet potato with olive oil and roast for 20 minutes.
3. In a skillet, sauté kale until wilted, about 3-4 minutes.
4. In the same skillet, fry the egg to your liking.
5. Assemble the bowl: Place kale at the bottom, then add roasted sweet potato.
6. Top with the fried egg, sliced avocado, and salsa.
7. Season with salt and pepper to taste.

My Notes:

_____

_____

_____

Sheet Pan Chicken Fajitas (Dinner)

Serving Size: 2 fajitas

Nutritional Information (approximate):

Calories: 400
Carbohydrates: 35g
Fat: 18g
Sugar: 5g

Ingredients:

- 6 oz (170g) chicken breast, sliced
- 1 bell pepper, sliced
- 1/2 onion, sliced
- 1 tbsp (15ml) olive oil
- 2 tsp fajita seasoning
- 2 small whole-wheat tortillas
- 2 tbsp (30g) salsa
- 2 tbsp (30g) guacamole

Directions:

1. Preheat oven to 425°F (220°C).
2. In a bowl, toss chicken, bell pepper, and onion with olive oil and fajita seasoning.
3. Spread mixture on a baking sheet in a single layer.
4. Roast for 15-20 minutes, stirring once halfway through.
5. Warm tortillas in the oven for the last minute.
6. Serve chicken and vegetables in tortillas, topped with salsa and guacamole.

My Notes:

_____

_____

_____

_____

Shrimp Stir-Fry with Brown Rice (Dinner)

Serving Size: 1 cup stir-fry with 1/2 cup cooked brown rice

Nutritional Information (approximate):

Calories: 380
Carbohydrates: 45g
Fat: 10g
Sugar: 4g

Ingredients:

- 4 oz (115g) raw shrimp, peeled and deveined
- 1/2 cup (50g) broccoli florets
- 1/4 cup (35g) bell pepper, sliced
- 1/4 cup (30g) carrot, sliced
- 1/2 cup (85g) cooked brown rice
- 1 tbsp vegetable oil
- 1 clove garlic, minced
- 1 tsp grated ginger

For the sauce:

- 1 tbsp soy sauce
- 1 tsp sesame oil
- 1 tsp cornstarch
- 2 tbsp water
- 1 tsp honey

Directions:

1. Mix sauce ingredients in a small bowl.
2. Heat oil in a wok or large skillet over medium-high heat.
3. Add garlic and ginger, stir-fry for 30 seconds.
4. Add shrimp, cook for 1-2 minutes until pink.
5. Add vegetables, stir-fry for 2-3 minutes until crisp-tender.
6. Pour in sauce, cook for 1 minute until thickened.
7. Serve over brown rice, sprinkled with sesame seeds if desired.

My Notes:

Sliced Pear with Blue Cheese and Walnuts (Snack)

Serving Size: 1 medium pear with toppings

Nutritional Information (approximate):

Calories: 220
Carbohydrates: 30g
Fat: 12g
Sugar: 19g

Ingredients:

- 1 medium pear
- 1 oz (28g) blue cheese, crumbled
- 1 tbsp (7g) chopped walnuts
- 1 tsp honey (optional)

Directions:

1. Wash and slice the pear into 8-10 wedges.
2. Arrange pear slices on a plate.
3. Sprinkle crumbled blue cheese over the pear slices.
4. Top with chopped walnuts.
5. If desired, drizzle with honey.
6. Serve immediately.

My Notes:

_____

_____

_____

_____

Slow Cooker Turkey Chili Serving (Dinner)

Size: 1 cup (240ml) chili

Nutritional Information (approximate):

Calories: 250
Carbohydrates: 30g
Fat: 8g
Sugar: 5g

Ingredients:

- 1 lb (450g) lean ground turkey
- 1 can (14.5 oz/411g) diced tomatoes
- 1 can (15 oz/425g) black beans, drained and rinsed
- 1 cup (150g) frozen corn
- 1 medium onion, diced
- 1 bell pepper, diced
- 2 cloves garlic, minced
- 2 tbsp chili powder
- 1 tsp ground cumin
- 1 tsp dried oregano
- 1/2 tsp salt
- 1/4 tsp black pepper
- 1 cup (240ml) low-sodium chicken broth

For serving (optional):

- 1/4 cup (28g) shredded cheddar cheese
- 1 small piece of cornbread

Directions:

1. In a large skillet over medium heat, brown the ground turkey, breaking it up with a spoon.
2. Transfer the cooked turkey to the slow cooker.
3. Add diced tomatoes, black beans, corn, onion, bell pepper, and garlic to the slow cooker.
4. Stir in chili powder, cumin, oregano, salt, and pepper.
5. Pour in the chicken broth and stir to combine all ingredients.
6. Cover and cook on low for 6-8 hours, or on high for 3-4 hours.
7. Taste and adjust seasoning if needed.
8. Serve hot, topped with shredded cheese if desired, with a side of cornbread.

Note: This recipe makes approximately 6 servings. Leftovers can be stored in an airtight container in the refrigerator for up to 3 days or frozen for up to 3 months.

Spaghetti Squash with Marinara and Meatballs (Dinner)

Serving Size: 1 cup squash with sauce and 3 meatballs

Nutritional Information (approximate):

Calories: 350
Carbohydrates: 30g
Fat: 18g
Sugar: 10g

Ingredients:

- 1/2 medium spaghetti squash (about 600g)
- 1/2 cup (120ml) marinara sauce
- 3 turkey meatballs (about 90g)
- 1 tbsp (5g) grated Parmesan cheese
- Salt and pepper to taste

Directions:

1. Preheat oven to 400°F (200°C).
2. Cut spaghetti squash in half lengthwise and scoop out seeds.
3. Place cut-side down on a baking sheet and roast for 40-45 minutes until tender.
4. While squash is roasting, heat marinara sauce and meatballs in a saucepan.
5. Once squash is done, use a fork to scrape the flesh into spaghetti-like strands.
6. Top squash with marinara and meatballs, sprinkle with Parmesan cheese.
7. Season with salt and pepper to taste.

My Notes:

_____

_____

_____

_____

Superfood Smoothie Bowl (Breakfast)

Serving Size: 1 bowl (approximately 2 cups or 16 fl oz)

Nutritional Information (per serving):

Calories: 350
Carbohydrates: 45g
Fat: 12g
Sugar: 25g

Ingredients (for 1 serving):

- 1 cup frozen mixed berries
- 1/2 medium ripe banana (about 1/2 cup sliced)
- 1 cup fresh spinach, loosely packed
- 3/4 cup unsweetened almond milk
- 1 scoop (30g) vanilla protein powder

For topping:

- 1 tbsp sliced almonds
- 1 tsp chia seeds
- 1 tsp honey

Directions:

1. In a blender, combine the frozen berries, banana, spinach, almond milk, and protein powder.
2. Blend on high speed until smooth and creamy, about 30-45 seconds. If the mixture is too thick, add a little more almond milk, 1 tablespoon at a time.
3. Pour the smoothie mixture into a bowl.
4. Top with sliced almonds and chia seeds.
5. Drizzle honey over the top.
6. Serve immediately and enjoy your nutrient-packed Superfood Smoothie Bowl!

My Notes:

_____

_____

_____

Stuffed Portobello Mushrooms (Dinner)

Serving Size: 2 stuffed mushroom caps

Nutritional Information (approximate):

Calories: 280
Carbohydrates: 25g
Fat: 18g
Sugar: 4g

Ingredients:

- 2 large portobello mushroom caps
- 1/2 cup (85g) cooked quinoa
- 1 cup (30g) fresh spinach
- 2 tbsp (30g) feta cheese, crumbled
- 1 tbsp olive oil
- 1 clove garlic, minced
- Salt and pepper to taste

Directions:

1. Preheat oven to 375°F (190°C).
2. Remove stems from mushrooms and gently scrape out gills.
3. In a skillet, heat olive oil and sauté garlic and spinach until wilted.
4. Mix sautéed spinach with quinoa and feta cheese.
5. Fill mushroom caps with the mixture.
6. Place on a baking sheet and bake for 20-25 minutes until mushrooms are tender.

My Notes:

_____

_____

_____

_____

Sweet Potato Toast with Avocado (Breakfast)

Serving Size: 2 slices

Nutritional Information (approximate):

Calories: 250
Carbohydrates: 35g
Fat: 14g
Sugar: 6g

Ingredients:

- 1 medium sweet potato
- 1/2 ripe avocado
- 1/4 tsp sea salt
- 1 tsp hot sauce
- 1 tsp olive oil

Directions:

1. Wash and slice sweet potato lengthwise into 1/4-inch thick slices.
2. Brush slices with olive oil.
3. Toast sweet potato slices in a toaster or under the broiler for 5-7 minutes per side, until tender.
4. Mash avocado in a small bowl.
5. Spread mashed avocado on sweet potato slices.
6. Sprinkle with sea salt and drizzle with hot sauce.
7. Serve immediately.

My Notes:

_____

_____

_____

_____

Tuna Salad Lettuce Wraps (Lunch)

Serving Size: 2 lettuce wraps

Nutritional Information (approximate):

Calories: 220
Carbohydrates: 6g
Fat: 10g
Sugar: 2g

Ingredients:

- 1 can (5 oz/142g) tuna in water, drained
- 2 tbsp (30g) Greek yogurt
- 1/4 cup (30g) celery, finely diced
- 2 tbsp (20g) red onion, finely diced
- 2 large lettuce leaves (romaine or butter lettuce)
- 1/2 lemon, juiced
- Salt and pepper to taste

Directions:

1. In a bowl, mix tuna, Greek yogurt, celery, and red onion.
2. Season with salt and pepper to taste.
3. Wash and dry lettuce leaves.
4. Spoon the tuna mixture onto the lettuce leaves.
5. Squeeze lemon juice over the top.
6. Serve immediately.

My Notes:

_____

_____

_____

_____

Turkey and Avocado Wrap (Lunch)

Serving Size: 1 wrap

Nutritional Information (approximate):

Calories: 420
Carbohydrates: 35g
Fat: 23g
Sugar: 4g

Ingredients:

- 1 large (10-inch) whole-grain wrap
- 2 tbsp (30g) hummus
- 3 oz (85g) sliced turkey breast
- 1/4 medium avocado, sliced (about 50g)
- 1 large leaf of romaine lettuce
- 2 slices of tomato (about 30g)
- Salt and pepper to taste

Directions:

1. Lay the whole-grain wrap flat on a clean surface.
2. Spread the hummus evenly over the entire surface of the wrap, leaving a small border around the edges.
3. Layer the sliced turkey breast in the center of the wrap, covering about 2/3 of the surface.
4. Arrange the avocado slices on top of the turkey.
5. Place the lettuce leaf over the avocado.
6. Add the tomato slices on top of the lettuce.
7. Sprinkle with salt and pepper to taste.
8. To roll the wrap, fold in both sides over the filling.
9. Starting from the end closest to you, tightly roll the wrap away from you, enclosing all the ingredients.
10. Cut the wrap diagonally in half for easier eating.
11. Serve immediately or wrap in foil or parchment paper for a portable lunch.

My Notes:

_____

_____

Turkey-Zucchini Meatballs with Spaghetti (Dinner)

Serving Size: 4 meatballs with 1 cup cooked spaghetti

Nutritional Information (approximate):

Calories: 420
Carbohydrates: 55g
Fat: 12g
Sugar: 8g

Ingredients:

- 8 oz (225g) ground turkey
- 1/2 cup (50g) grated zucchini
- 1/4 cup (30g) breadcrumbs
- 2 tbsp (10g) grated Parmesan cheese
- 1 egg
- 1 clove garlic, minced
- 2 oz (56g) whole-grain spaghetti, dry
- 1/2 cup (120ml) marinara sauce
- Salt and pepper to taste

Directions:

1. Preheat oven to 375°F (190°C).
2. In a bowl, mix turkey, zucchini, breadcrumbs, Parmesan, egg, garlic, salt, and pepper.
3. Form mixture into 4 meatballs.
4. Place meatballs on a baking sheet and bake for 20-25 minutes until cooked through.
5. Meanwhile, cook spaghetti according to package instructions.
6. Heat marinara sauce in a saucepan.
7. Serve meatballs over spaghetti and top with marinara sauce.

My Notes:

_____

_____

_____

Veggie-Hummus Wrap (Lunch)

Serving Size: 1 wrap

Nutritional Information (approximate):

Calories: 320
Carbohydrates: 40g
Fat: 15g
Sugar: 5g

Ingredients:

- 1 large whole-grain wrap
- 3 tbsp (45g) hummus
- 1/4 cup (30g) cucumber, sliced
- 1/4 cup (30g) bell pepper, sliced
- 1/4 cup (25g) carrot, shredded
- 1/2 cup (15g) lettuce leaves

Directions:

1. Lay the wrap flat on a clean surface.
2. Spread hummus evenly over the wrap, leaving a small border around the edges.
3. Layer cucumber, bell pepper, carrot, and lettuce over the hummus.
4. Fold in both sides of the wrap over the filling.
5. Starting from one end, tightly roll up the wrap.
6. Cut in half diagonally and serve.

My Notes:

Veggie-Packed Frittata (Lunch)

Serving Size: 1/4 of frittata (approximately 1 large slice)

Nutritional Information (approximate):

Calories: 220
Carbohydrates: 6g
Fat: 16g
Sugar: 3g

Ingredients:

- 6 large eggs
- 2 tbsp (30ml) milk
- 1 tbsp (15ml) olive oil
- 1 cup (30g) fresh spinach, roughly chopped
- 1/2 cup (50g) mushrooms, sliced
- 1/4 cup (35g) bell peppers, diced
- 1/4 cup (25g) shredded cheese (cheddar or mozzarella)
- Salt and pepper to taste

Directions:

1. Preheat oven to 375°F (190°C).
2. In a large bowl, whisk together eggs, milk, salt, and pepper. Set aside.
3. Heat olive oil in a 10-inch oven-safe skillet over medium heat.
4. Add mushrooms and bell peppers to the skillet. Sauté for 3-4 minutes until softened.
5. Add spinach and cook until wilted, about 1-2 minutes.
6. Spread the vegetables evenly in the skillet.
7. Pour the egg mixture over the vegetables, tilting the pan to distribute evenly.
8. Cook on the stovetop for 3-4 minutes, until the edges start to set.
9. Sprinkle the shredded cheese evenly over the top.
10. Transfer the skillet to the preheated oven.
11. Bake for 10-12 minutes, or until the frittata is set and lightly golden on top.
12. Remove from the oven and let cool for 5 minutes.
13. Slice into quarters and serve warm.

My Notes:

Veggie-Packed Minestrone Soup (Lunch)

Serving Size: 1 bowl (approximately 1.5 cups or 350 ml)

Nutritional Information (approximate):

Calories: 220
Carbohydrates: 35g
Fat: 6g
Sugar: 8g

Ingredients:

- 1/2 cup (120ml) diced tomatoes
- 1/4 cup (30g) zucchini, diced
- 1/4 cup (30g) carrot, diced
- 1/4 cup (30g) celery, diced
- 1/4 cup (45g) canned white beans, drained and rinsed
- 1 cup (240ml) vegetable broth
- 1/2 cup (15g) fresh spinach
- 1 tbsp (5g) grated Parmesan cheese
- 1 tsp olive oil
- 1 small garlic clove, minced
- 1/4 tsp dried basil
- Salt and pepper to taste

Directions:

1. In a pot, heat olive oil over medium heat. Add garlic and sauté for 30 seconds.
2. Add carrots and celery, cook for 3-4 minutes.
3. Add zucchini, tomatoes, beans, broth, and basil. Bring to a boil.
4. Reduce heat and simmer for 15-20 minutes until vegetables are tender.
5. Stir in spinach and cook for another 2 minutes.
6. Season with salt and pepper to taste.
7. Serve hot, topped with grated Parmesan cheese.

My Notes:

Zucchini Noodles with Pesto and Chicken (Dinner)

Serving Size: 1 bowl (approximately 2 cups)

Nutritional Information (approximate):

Calories: 350
Carbohydrates: 12g
Fat: 22g
Sugar: 5g

Ingredients:

- 2 medium zucchini (about 14 oz/400g)
- 4 oz (115g) grilled chicken breast, sliced
- 2 tbsp (30g) homemade or store-bought pesto
- 1/2 cup (75g) cherry tomatoes, halved
- 1 tbsp (5g) grated Parmesan cheese
- Salt and pepper to taste

For homemade pesto (makes extra):

- 2 cups fresh basil leaves
- 2 cloves garlic
- 1/4 cup (35g) pine nuts
- 1/2 cup (120ml) olive oil
- 1/4 cup (25g) grated Parmesan cheese
- Salt to taste

Directions:

1. If making homemade pesto, blend basil, garlic, and pine nuts in a food processor. Slowly add olive oil while blending.
2. Stir in Parmesan cheese and salt.
3. Spiralize the zucchini into noodles using a spiralizer or vegetable peeler.
4. In a large bowl, toss the zucchini noodles with 2 tablespoons of pesto until evenly coated.
5. Heat a large non-stick skillet over medium heat.
6. Add the zucchini noodles to the skillet and cook for 2-3 minutes, until just tender.
7. Transfer the warm zucchini noodles to a serving bowl.
8. Top with sliced grilled chicken breast.
9. Add halved cherry tomatoes.
10. Sprinkle grated Parmesan cheese over the top.
11. Season with salt and pepper to taste.
12. Serve immediately while still warm.xf

INDEX OF MOVEMENTS

Index of Movements

REFERENCES

AceFitness. (2017, April 19). *Meal timing: What and when to eat for performance and recovery*. Ace Fitness. https://www.acefitness.org/resources/pros/expert-articles/6390/meal-timing-what-and-when-to-eat-for-performance-and-recovery/

Agnes. (2023, March 7). *Structure and alignment*: Acudragon Wellness System. https://acudragonnyc.com/index.php/2023/03/07/

Chao, A. M., Jastreboff, A. M., White, M. A., Grilo, C. M., & Sinha, R. (2017). *Stress, cortisol, and other appetite-related hormones: Prospective prediction of 6-month changes in food cravings and weight*. Obesity, 25(4), 713–720. https://doi.org/10.1002/oby.21790

Cronkleton, E. (2019, July 12). *6 warm-up exercises to help boost your workout*. Healthline; Healthline Media. https://www.healthline.com/health/fitness-exercise/warm-up-exercises

Dudley, C. (2019, November 13). *Touch as a feedback mechanism for athletes*. Elite FTS. https://www.elitefts.com/education/touch-as-a-feedback-mechanism-for-athletes/

Gunnars, K. (2019, June 7). *27 health and nutrition tips that are actually evidence-based*. Healthline; Healthline Media. https://www.healthline.com/nutrition/27-health-and-nutrition-tips

Karadsheh, S. (2020, December 28). *Top 25 Mediterranean recipes to try in 2021*. The Mediterranean Dish. https://www.themediterraneandish.com/best-mediterranean-recipes-of-2018/

National Institute of Health. (2018, April 4). *The benefits of slumber*. NIH News in Health; U.S. Department of Health and Human Services. https://newsinhealth.nih.gov/2013/04/benefits-slumber

Olive Content Team. (n.d.). *35 Mediterranean recipes*. Olivemagazine. https://www.olivemagazine.com/recipes/collection/best-mediterranean-recipes/

Pilates Foundation Team. (n.d.). *About Pilates | Pilates Foundation*. Www.Pilatesfoundation.com. https://www.Pilatesfoundation.com/about-Pilates

Rishe, A. (2024, March 6). *How to maintain a healthy lifestyle: 12 effective tips*. Healthline. https://www.healthline.com/health/how-to-maintain-a-healthy-lifestyle

Weir, K. (2020, April 1). Nurtured by nature. *American Psychological Association, 51*(3), 50. https://www.apa.org/monitor/2020/04/nurtured-nature

Yamato, T. P., Maher, C. G., Saragiotto, B. T., Hancock, M. J., Ostelo, R. W. J. G., Cabral, C. M. N., Costa, L. C. M., & Costa, L. O. P. (2016). Pilates for Low Back Pain. *SPINE, 41*(12), 1013–1021. https://doi.org/10.1097/brs.0000000000001398

www.ingramcontent.com/pod-product-compliance
Lightning Source LLC
Chambersburg PA
CBHW080419030426

42335CB00020B/2509